# Praise For: *Cancer & The Biology Of Hope*

"This book is a lifeline for those who feel lost in the chaos of a cancer diagnosis. Dr. Lemmon offers not just information, but inspiration, showing patients how to move from fear to hope and from illness to healing. *Cancer & The Biology of Hope* invites every reader to become the hero of their own healing story."

– **Dr. Nalini Chilkov**, Founder, OutSmart Cancer®, American Institute of Integrative Oncology, Author *32 Ways to OutSmart Cancer: How to Create A Body Where Cancer Cannot Thrive*

"Dr. David Lemmon's book, *Cancer and the Biology of Hope: The 7 Pathways of Healing*, is a heartfelt and comprehensive guide to integrative cancer care written by a doctor with a great depth of compassion and expertise. If you or someone you love is seeking a book to take along on a cancer healing journey I would highly recommend *Cancer and the Biology of Hope* as an inspiring and empowering resource to help light the way."

– **Mark Bricca, ND, LAc** Owner at Bodhicitta Healing Arts

"*Cancer and the Biology of Hope* is a masterpiece. It is a must-read in today's environment of ever-increasing cancer incidence, toxins in our environment and even in our food, and near panic in the face of a diagnosis. It is a courageous book, demonstrating how nonmedical and medical approaches are not contradictory but rather can offer complementary options for each person who must make choices for themselves or a loved one. Dr. Lemmon's explanations of the basic science of cancer and the body's response to it are refreshingly clear and on target. His comprehensive, up-to-date review of all the major modalities in his seven pathways of healing leaves no stone unturned. And his emphasis on hope and healing is a true gift. If you have any concerns about cancer, this is the book you want."

–**Randy Rolfe**, author of The Single Ingredient Diet: Transform Your Relationship to Food in 21 Days. https://singleingredientdiet.com/freeworkshop

"*Cancer & The Biology of Hope* is a beacon of clarity, compassion, and empowerment. Dr. Lemmon masterfully bridges science and soul, offering a deeply holistic path forward for those navigating cancer. This book is a must-have for anyone seeking true healing—not just physically, but emotionally and spiritually. I'll be recommending this to my clients and community."

— **Paula Sherrill**, Holistic Health Coach & Founder of Sher Essentials & The Wellness Impact Movement   empwrlife.com/dc/512/330360

"*Cancer & The Biology of Hope* by Dr. David Lemmon is a groundbreaking guide that redefines how we understand and approach cancer. More than just a medical condition, cancer is a whole-life challenge — and healing requires a whole-person response. Blending modern science, ancient wisdom, and years of clinical insight, Dr. Lemmon introduces *The 7 Pathways of Healing* — a transformative framework that empowers patients, caregivers, and those seeking prevention. This book delivers more than information; it offers resilience, clarity, and real hope on every step of the journey."

–**Tavares A. Garrett**    Author of *The Body Synthesis*

"Dr. Lemmon knows better than most that the body is a self-healing miracle. And he knows what the body needs in order to be able to heal. This book will show you those healing pathways."

— **Bob Ross, EMT-D**   TheHiddenSecretToHealing.com

"As a person that looks for holistic approaches first to heal my body, *Cancer & The Biology of Hope* would be the first thing that I would read if ever diagnosed with the horrible disease of Cancer. I have heard of people beating Cancer using holistic practices but I didn't know how. This book provides a great foundation to understand that there are alternative options that work. Thank you Dr. Lemmon for sharing your work with the world and truly making a difference!"

— **Kellie Rhymes**   Limitless Mindset Coaching   www.limitlessmindsetcoach.com

"This insightful work navigates the complex journey of cancer treatment and recovery, merging scientific understanding with a profound sense of optimism.

Dr. Lemmon masterfully delineates seven essential pathways that empower patients and caregivers alike. His compassionate narrative combines personal stories and scientific research, making it accessible and engaging for readers from all walks of life.

Whether you are a patient, a healthcare professional, or someone seeking to understand the healing journey. Dr. Lemmon's expertise and empathetic approach shine through, making *Cancer and the Biology of Hope* an essential read for anyone touched by cancer. Highly recommended!"

–Therese Forton-Barnes  The Low-Tox Living Guru   https://thegreenlivinggurus.com/

"In *Cancer & The Biology of Hope: The 7 Pathways of Healing*, Dr. David Lemmon has uniquely combined his knowledge, experience with patients, and research into a guidebook for those seeking the beneficial journey with cancer to new possibilities of healing in mind, body, and spirit. He aptly quotes Norman Cousins and firmly believes this statement: "Each patient carries his own doctor inside him." Let us all believe that too. He empowers readers with hope throughout and cheers them on through every chapter of this book. Fear-inducing beliefs are shattered and the paths become clearer. By following the seven pathways that he introduces to you, with emphasis on choices that always align with your unique being, you will be transforming, healing, and enriching your world. Many of the therapies are free or cost close to nothing. The resources are immense. This book can be used both as a reference and as a workbook. It will serve you the best if you allow it to inspire you into action. Being familiar with many of the therapies mentioned, I was saying, "Yes, yes, yes!" throughout, applauding the exposition of all this information. I must say

that this book added some tasty ingredients to my soup of knowledge, especially in the integrative healing realm."

– **Stacey-Anne Bistak**,   Certified Holistic Nutritionist and Lifestyle Practitioner  https://www.fernzholisticconsulting.com

# Cancer & The Biology of Hope: The 7 Pathways of Healing

Everything You Need To Know.
The Doctor's & Patient's Guide to Holistic Cancer Care,
Reducing the Side Effects of Chemo & Radiation,
Diet, Prevention, Long-Term Remission Support,
& Dramatically Enhancing Quality of Life.

By Dr David Lemmon

**Revive Publishing**

Vancouver, WA U.S.A.

Copyright 2025 by Dr David Lemmon

All rights reserved.

**Disclaimer:**

The information presented in this book is intended for educational and informational purposes only. It is not a substitute for professional medical advice, diagnosis, or treatment. The author does not claim to offer medical advice, nor does he recommend self-management of health problems without the guidance of qualified healthcare professionals.

This book discusses holistic and integrative approaches to cancer care, including both conventional and natural lifestyle approaches. Readers are strongly advised to consult with their oncologist, primary care physician, and licensed natural healthcare provider before beginning any new treatment regimen, altering current medications, or making decisions regarding the direction of their medical care.

The approaches described in this book may not be appropriate for all individuals or all types and stages of cancer. Every patient is unique, and cancer treatment should be personalized under the supervision of a qualified medical team. While efforts have been made to ensure the accuracy of the content, the field of medicine is constantly evolving, and new information may become available that could affect the interpretations of the information provided here.

The author and publishers disclaim any liability for any adverse effects, loss, or injury caused directly or indirectly from the use of information contained in this book.

**To Natalie**

I wish we had more time together on earth.

Thank you for the memories, and for your smile, love, courage, and inspiration to so many.

# Contents

Foreword- by Donnie Yance ..................................................................................8

Introduction ...........................................................................................................11

Chapter 1- Your Hero's Healing Journey ..........................................................22

Chapter 2- Introducing The 7 Pathways of Healing for Cancer ...................26

Chapter 3- Four Major Goals of Natural Healing ..........................................33

Chapter 4- Basic Concepts About Cancer ........................................................38

Chapter 5- The Emotional Pathway ..................................................................45

Chapter 6- The Energetic Pathway ....................................................................55

Chapter 7- The Molecular Pathway: Part 1- Food ..........................................63

Chapter 8- The Molecular Pathway: Part 2- Herbal Medicine .....................82

Chapter 9- The Molecular Pathway: Part 3- Supplements ..........................113

Chapter 10- The Molecular Pathway: Part 4- Mushrooms & Oils .............157

Chapter 11- The Molecular Pathway: Part 5- Lab Testing ..........................172

Chapter 12- The Molecular Pathway: Part 6- Molecules to Avoid ............180

Chapter 13- The Physical Pathway: Part 1- Exercise, Breath, & Fasting ..............184

Chapter 14- The Physical Pathway: Part 2- Other Physical Treatments ................190

Chapter 15- The Genetic Pathway ...................................................................196

Chapter 16- The Social Pathway ......................................................................203

Chapter 17- The Spiritual Pathway .................................................................206

Chapter 18- If You Undergo Surgery, Chemotherapy, or Radiation ..................218

# Foreword

When you or someone you love hears those three devastating words—"you have cancer"—time seems to stop.

In that moment, you join millions of others who have faced this challenge, each with their own unique story of struggle, courage, and ultimately, hope.

Over my four decades providing global support for cancer patients through the Mederi Care methodology, I've witnessed countless individuals embark on this journey, often overwhelmed by clinical jargon, contradictory advice, pervasive misinformation online, and the pressure to make life-altering decisions quickly. Too often, they're presented with a narrow path focused solely on conventional treatments, leaving them wondering if they're missing critical elements of healing.

A whole systems approach to cancer, such as Mederi Care, challenges the current reductionistic health care system, not by being *against* anything, but being *for* something even better. By focusing on what we're for rather than what we're against, we create space for collaboration rather than confrontation. This approach invites participation from diverse stakeholders—patients, practitioners, researchers, and communities—in the co-creation of healthcare that truly serves human flourishing.

Dr. David Lemmon's comprehensive guide fills this gap beautifully. What makes "Cancer & The Biology of Hope" truly exceptional is its balanced, holistic approach that respects both conventional medicine and complementary therapies. This isn't about choosing sides in the false dichotomy between "traditional" and "alternative" medicine—it's about integration, or better yet, "unification"—as well as personalization and wholeness.

The 7 Pathways framework offers something rare in medical literature: a truly comprehensive roadmap that addresses not just the physical aspects of cancer treatment, but the emotional, energetic, molecular, genetic, social, and spiritual dimensions equally vital to healing. These various networks are all interconnected, and when we support this interconnection rather than fragmenting our approach, we enable true healing. This isn't merely theoretical—it's practical, actionable wisdom drawn from both rigorous research and years of clinical experience.

Conventional modern medicine has long separated itself from traditional healing systems such as Traditional Chinese Medicine, Ayurveda, and the Eclectic tradition. However, the inadequacies of conventional medicine and the growing interest of people in the wisdom of these ancient healing traditions has created a unique opportunity to rewrite medicine as we currently know it. I believe the time is now ripe for a truly holistic medical approach to emerge.

What resonates most powerfully throughout these pages is an underlying current of hope—not the false hope of miracle cures or unrealistic promises, but the authentic hope that comes from empowerment, informed choice, and the recognition that healing occurs on multiple levels. Dr. Lemmon reminds us that while we cannot control everything about cancer, we can control how we respond to it, and that response can dramatically impact not just survival, but quality of life.

I am guided by Ben Franklin's brilliant insight: *"A place for everything, and everything its place."*

I strongly believe that the foundation of health is rooted in herbal remedies, nutrition, dietary choices, lifestyle therapies, and spiritual nourishment.

As Andy Dufresne reminds us, *"Hope is a good thing, maybe the best of things, and no good thing ever dies."*

Rachel Naomi Remen beautifully articulates in *The Gray Zone*, *"The wish to control floats like a buoy above the hidden reef of fear. More than any single thing, fear is the stumbling block to life's agenda. Perhaps it is only the things we fear that we wish to control. No one can serve life if they are unconsciously afraid of life."*

Rather than living in fear, we have the ability to cultivate both optimism and hope. Pope Francis distinguishes between the two:

*"It is useful not to confuse optimism and hope. Optimism is a psychological attitude to life. Hope goes further; it is an anchor thrown to the future, which allows one to pull on its rope to arrive at the goal one longs for, by using our*

*effort to move in the right direction. In addition, hope is theological: God is there in the middle of it. For all these reasons, I believe that life is going to triumph."*

Whether you're a patient seeking options beyond what your oncologist has offered, a caregiver looking to support a loved one, or a healthcare practitioner hoping to expand your understanding of integrative cancer care, this book offers invaluable guidance for the journey ahead. It stands as a testament to the power of approaching cancer with both cutting-edge science and timeless healing wisdom.

May these pages bring you not just information, but transformation—and above all, the courage to embrace hope as an essential element of your healing journey.

With deep respect for your path,

**Donnie Yance**  CN MH RH(AHG)


Donnie is the best-selling author of *Herbal Medicine, Healing & Cancer* and *Adaptogens in Medical Herbalism*. He is the founder of the Mederi Center Clinic and Natura Health Products. You can explore hundreds of his health posts at www.donnieyance.com

# Introduction

"You have cancer."

These are among the most feared 3 words In the English language.

What happens next can be dizzying...

the overwhelm, the fear,

the questions, the confusion...

Why me?

Why now?

Is this the end?

What should I do?

Who should I turn to?

Your life gets derailed in a single moment, and it can be hard to see light at the end of this tunnel.

I know it's devastating, and the pain is real. While I cannot change that, my hope is that with this book you will gain the methods to keep that light of hope always shining brightly into the future.

There are many who have walked this healing journey before you, and their voices beckon you onward.

If they could speak with a collective voice, they might say that,

"It's possible to reduce the side effects of conventional treatments like: nausea, vomiting, brain fog, fatigue, hair loss, and pain, and at the same time boost the effectiveness of chemo and radiation."

You may have heard (and maybe cringed!) that some patients have said,

"Cancer is the best thing that ever happened to me."

Why would anyone in their right mind say something like that?

Because if you go about cancer treatments in a holistic integrative way...

It's possible to emerge on the other side of your cancer journey feeling even *happier and healthier* than ever before. Cancer can rearrange your priorities, and alert you to life's 'blind spots' like nothing else.

By going through this transformational 7 Pathways process...

You can come away with increased feelings of peace, well-being, confidence, joy, and balance in nearly *every* area of your life.

You can make your conventional cancer treatments *more* effective...

and improve your health, energy, stress levels, mood, relationships, goals, and spiritual life at the *same* time.

It's time to treat cancer in a way that combines the very best of cutting-edge science along with time-tested healing knowledge.

Sound good?

Then let's get started....

## I Believe In You

First off, I want you to know that I believe in you and your body's innate healing capacity. I know you can do hard things, amazing things, and even so-called 'impossible' things. You are a warrior of light: strong beyond measure, powerful beyond understanding, and wise beyond words. It's your human birthright. You may not see it or recognize it all the time, but it's in there; in your Soul, your unconquerable Spirit, your Heart, and your Mind.

You are a *hero*. All the great stories of myth, book, and film are great because they are about *you*. These stories remind us who we truly are inside, and who we know deep down that we can one day become. As a human race, we have inherited this hidden hero's DNA from all of our innumerable ancestors that have overcome, survived, and thrived through all the generations of time.

## Why I wrote this book

In September 2012, my younger sister Natalie went into the emergency room with shortness of breath and rapid heart beat. They told her to follow up with her primary care doctor, which she did. They did some blood work, and were looking for the possibility of a blood clot. They did a scan for the blood clot, and they instead saw two spots on her liver, which they were concerned about.

They scheduled her for a CT scan of all her organs, and the report came back with 5 masses on her liver. The doctor told Natalie that it looked like liver cancer. After a biopsy, it was found to be a rare form of bile-duct cancer that had already spread to her liver.

Her oncologist called her in and said, "I'm sorry.... but you have a 0% chance of survival."

Meanwhile, I was several states away in the middle of my naturopathic medical school program. I was learning about all the amazing remedies, treatments, and options available for cancer support. But I didn't have the time or money to fly out and visit her, so we talked on the phone a few times..

I thought we would have more time. I thought there would be more opportunities to research, to share, to laugh, to live.

But only 6 weeks later, she was gone...

This beautiful, apparently healthy, young woman in her early 30's left behind a husband and 2 young children.

I never got to say goodbye; and I didn't get to see her until the funeral. It shattered my heart into millions of tiny pieces. So this event lit a fire inside my soul. I was filled with a consuming passion to *never* let anyone else go through this kind of challenge without having answers at their fingertips. Lots of answers...

I have dedicated the past 15 years of my life to studying cancer; what causes it, and what reverses it. Since then, I've worked with thousands of patients, and now I'm excited to share this experience with you.

I believe this is one of the most comprehensive books on holistic cancer care ever published. My research team and I have delved into over 1,000 medical studies, sifted through hundreds of hours of medical training, and have compiled the best solutions from all around the world into one powerful life-changing resource.

A blend of science and art, tradition and cutting-edge technology, this book is my life's work. It is infused with love, and dedicated to the memory of my beloved sister. I love you Nat!

## Transforming and Transcending

I believe that one of the great purposes of life is to transcend our limitations and become the best version of ourselves that we can. This process of transformation is very often a painful one, but as we expand our vision, we can know that it is all worth it in the end.

A caterpillar may experience discomfort and claustrophobia encased, even buried alive, suffocating in its chrysalis. The experience of darkness and constriction transforms it. It becomes a new creature; with more abilities, freedom, beauty, and color than ever before. This is *your* destiny too.

In the ancient process of refining gold, raw ore was heated to burn off impurities. The dregs, all the unwanted crud, was scraped away until nothing remained but the beautiful, pure, glorious, 'golden' gold. It was now ready to shine as a symbol of gods and kings, and one of the very definitions of ultimate wealth. But the burning and the scraping, the fire and the torment, are all too real when we're in these moments of maximum heat. This fire too shall pass; eventually the refiner's fire cools down, but the gold that you have become remains forever untarnished, shimmering in the sunlight.

Michelangelo faced a massive marble block that had been started and abandoned by at least 2 other Italian sculptors. This creamy white slab of Carrera marble was nicknamed 'Il Gigante' or 'The Giant' and was the starting point for one of the largest and most famous works of art in history. The stone block had a weird hole drilled through it, and it was cut in a strange shape. Michelangelo studied it, saw with his mind's eye the mighty figure concealed within, and went to work. Hammer and chisel pounding, pounding, pounding away; cutting, breaking, chipping, beating that poor marble to death. He kept on removing all that didn't belong to the perfection deep beneath the rough surface. We can imagine if the stone had feelings, it might have said, "Why won't it stop! I can't take it anymore, what did I do to deserve this? Just stop with the hammering, *please!*" But the lesson, of course, is that after the hammering, chipping, and polishing were done, Michelangelo's 'David' remained. Five hundred years later, it is still revered as one of the greatest sculptures of all time, and this 17-foot giant is visited by about 1.5 million people every year. Life is the hammer. We are the marble. God, Nature, and the Universe want to transform us into one of the greatest artworks of all time.

The choice is always the same; give up and become a statistic, or participate in the process of transformation to become a *masterpiece*.

What will you choose?

## Start With Happiness

Happiness is the ultimate goal for just about everything we set out to do.

- Why do you want to eat better and exercise? Because you think it will make you happy.

- Why do you spend years looking for the perfect romantic partner? Because you think it will make you happy.

- Why do you want to earn a million dollars? Because you think it will make you happy.

We often start at the wrong end when creating our goals, visualizations, and affirmations. We think we want weight loss, a perfect partner, or tons of cash. But what we really want is the happiness that we believe these things will bring.

So if you start at the wrong end, and just set out to eat right, go on lots of dates, or work 3 jobs, you might achieve these things, but there's no guarantee that you'll be happy with the results. Life works better when you put happiness first.

If you start with happiness as the goal, then from that place of happiness you can start to build a beautiful life. Things begin to flow from this place of joy, and it becomes easier to achieve all your other specific goals. In other words, if you start with happiness, you can then achieve health, romance, and wealth, and you know you'll be happy; But if you start chasing weight loss, relationships, or money, without first choosing to be happy, then you can be left unfulfilled and miserable even with your 6-pack abs, a 'trophy' partner, and a mansion on the hill.

This applies to a cancer diagnosis as well. If you start by choosing and cultivating happiness, then you can move on to more specific outcomes of health and healing. But if you just gear up for war and say, "we're going to beat this thing!" and then go full steam ahead to fight, battle, kill, or conquer the cancer, then you may or may not be happy for whatever years you have left.

If you start with happiness, then no matter what happens, you win! If the cancer grows more aggressive and you pass away within 6 months, then you had a happy, grateful, 6 months filled with life, joy, and love. If you happily follow and nurture the 7 Pathways of Healing and the cancer goes into a long-term remission, then you get to be happy *and* healthy for many years to come; But if you postpone happiness, and focus on only killing the tumor, then you can become stressed, miserable, and overwhelmed.

So choose happiness as your first goal. Then you can confidently and happily move down the 7 Pathways of Healing, knowing that no matter the outcome, you have already won.

## Freedom

One of the core principles of this book is *freedom*. I am a staunch advocate of medical freedom. You and I have the inalienable right to choose medical options that resonate with us personally, and the right to refuse medical care that we don't agree with. This also applies to parents' right to choose what they feel is the best medical care for their children, which unfortunately, is sometimes violated in violent ways.

But beyond medical freedom at the political level, this book is about options. You aren't free to choose an option that you don't know about, so education is the first step. This book is filled to the brim with options, and once you know about them you become *free* to act upon them. These options are shown to have powerful effects by scientific studies, long traditional use, or both.

You have the absolute right to use conventional medicine, natural medicine, or any combination of the two. This is your body and your life. These are decisions that can only be made in your own heart and mind with careful consultation with your healthcare team, and your closest family or friends. Be careful not to let well-meaning doctors, family members, or friends unduly sway your informed medical decisions. Chemo and radiation are clearly harmful and are proven to increase the risk of a future cancer recurrence, but it is the right path for many people. Trusting in natural medicine alone comes with its own set of risks, but it has helped many people as well. These issues are never black and white, and you should never allow yourself to be bullied or coerced into any treatment that you do not believe in and feel good about. Only you are fully entitled to receive inspiration and intuition for your own best healing journey.

Most of the information in this book is not yet known by medical schools, conventional doctors, or oncologists. That's why I wrote it; to get the word out to those who may not have easy access to integrative cancer centers, naturopathic oncology specialists, medical herbalists, or highly-trained holistic healers of any kind. I have done my absolute best to fill this book with truth, "and the truth shall make you *free*."

## Hope

This book is also about hope. The intangible world creates the tangible world, so the biology of hope takes into account the placebo effect; this is the most powerful and pure form of medicine there is. Belief in a positive outcome is the first step to aligning body, mind, and spirit for true healing. Some people worry about false hope, but 'having it' is what makes hope true. Hope is part of the medicine. You have to think, feel, believe, and hope that your body, mind, and spirit can heal from this challenge. If you, or a loved one, have been given any kind of prognosis that is negative, stressful, or hurtful, you can take it with a huge grain of salt. If, for example, you have been told that you have 6-12 months to live, you can recognize that this educated guess is based on statistics of people that have followed only conventional-standard-of-care treatments. If you read and follow this book, those statistics won't apply to you anymore. So you can just confidently step right over that 12-month 'deadline' like a kid stepping over a spider's web in the grass. Annoying, but no harm done. As long as you are breathing, there is *always* hope for you.

## How To Use This Book

The 7 Pathways are presented in no particular order. In crafting a comprehensive treatment plan, you may already be doing many things right. Those strong areas will need less attention. But the weaker pathways will need more urgent focus and action to become strong. So I have created this questionnaire to help you identify which pathways need the most attention, information, and action to fill in the gaps of your ideal treatment plan.

**Important note**- if you are in the middle of chemo or radiation treatments, or if you are considering surgery, chemo, or radiation, start by reading chapter 18. This will give you the integrative medicine strategies that you need to reduce side effects, prevent chemo resistance, target the chemo and radiation toward the cancer cells and away from your healthy cells, and heal better after surgery.

# The Questionnaire

(Circle the most correct answer for you right now.)

### The Emotional Pathway

My stress levels are calm and well managed.     **True / False**

I do not have any deep emotional traumas (accident, abuse, illness, job-loss, grief, divorce, etc) that I have not fully processed and healed from.     **True / False**

My thoughts are often positive, optimistic, and hopeful.     **True / False**

I have regular stress-relieving habits or hobbies in place.     **True / False**

I generally feel happy, and that life is good.     **True / False**

### The Energetic Pathway

I have tried acupuncture, reiki, or microcurrent medicine.     **True / False**

I try to limit my use of cell phones, wifi, and bluetooth devices.     **True / False**

I do not have a 'smart home' or smart meters for my home.     **True / False**

I try to use my cell phone close to my head for less than 20 minutes per day.     **True / False**

I do not get headaches, eye strain, or fatigue when I spend a long time in front of a computer, tablet, or phone.     **True / False**

### The Molecular Pathway

I avoid air fresheners, candles, dryer sheets, or cleaning chemicals around my home.     **True / False**

I buy and eat lots of organic fruits and vegetables.     **True / False**

I avoid processed, packaged, or fast foods whenever possible.     **True / False**

I have never smoked, chewed, or vaped tobacco products. **True / False**

I often use vitamins, supplements, or shop at a health food store. **True / False**

## The Physical Pathway

I get a lot of movement and exercise more than 3 days per week. **True / False**

I regularly get 7-9 hours of restful sleep. **True / False**

I practice deep belly breathing, or other relaxing breath work. **True / False**

I practice fasting or often take breaks from eating for more than 12 hours in a row. **True / False**

I get massages, go to a chiropractor, take relaxing baths, or do other physical self care practices on a regular basis. **True / False**

## The Genetic Pathway

I do not have more than 2 close relatives that have died of cancer. **True / False**

I have never tested positive for specific genetic cancer risk factors such as BRCA etc. **True / False**

I have never been told that I have precancerous lesions or polyps in the past. **True / False**

I have done genetic testing and I know something about my personal genetics. **True / False**

I have never had 2 close relatives who have been diagnosed with the same type of cancer. **True / False**

## The Social Pathway

I live with other family members or have a roommate that I like. **True / False**

I have a close friend or family member that can come to my doctor appointments with me. **True / False**

I feel socially connected and interact with others on a regular basis. **True / False**

I have a church, club, or team where I feel like I can belong. **True / False**

I am happy with my romantic relationship or lack thereof. **True / False**

**The Spiritual Pathway**

I have a set of spiritual practices that bring me joy (prayer, meditation, fasting, study, service, etc) **True / False**

I know my life's purpose and what makes me feel most alive. **True / False**

I have a written list of my personal values and goals. **True / False**

I strive to show gratitude, faith, and optimism through life's challenges. **True / False**

I feel a deep sense of connection to God, Nature, or the Universe. **True / False**

Scoring is easy. Add 1 point per 'True' answer. You can write your answers below.

|  | Score (0-5) | Priority Order (1-7) |
|---|---|---|
| The Emotional Pathway | ____ | ____ |
| The Energetic Pathway | ____ | ____ |
| The Molecular Pathway | ____ | ____ |
| The Physical Pathway | ____ | ____ |
| The Genetic Pathway | ____ | ____ |
| The Social Pathway | ____ | ____ |
| The Spiritual Pathway | ____ | ____ |

This evaluation is by no means perfect or complete, but it should give you a rough idea of how you are doing in each of the 7 Pathways.

Look at the scores in relation to each other. Order them in priority order with the lowest score first. Put a '1' next to the Pathway that needs the most attention (the lowest score). If there are Pathways with the same scores, just put the same number next to all of the Pathways that are tied.

How did you do?

**Are all of your answers high (4-5)?** That's great! This means you have a lot going for you, and this book will be about fine tuning your already healthy lifestyle and doing more deep detective work to figure out the root cause of the cancer.

**Are they all lower (0-3)?** No judgement, that just means there's lots of room for growth and adventure in the chapters ahead.

**Are they uneven (some high and some low)?** That means you have some areas that can use a lot of attention to bring your whole lifestyle into greater balance.

Alright, I hope you are getting excited!

Please read chapters 1-4 first to lay a solid foundation, then you can jump around the *Pathways* chapters depending on your scores and preferences.

We are going on a choose your own healing adventure starting now. With your priority order for reading and acting on the *Pathways* chapters in place, we are ready to move forward and awaken your hero within.

# Chapter 1

## Your Hero's Journey

"You are the hero of your own Story."

-Joseph Campbell

Joseph Campbell was a 20th-century author and scholar who dedicated his life to studying world mythology. Through his research, he discovered a common pattern underlying myths, legends, and epic tales across different cultures and time periods. This pattern has been called the "hero's journey", a narrative structure that outlines the transformation of an ordinary individual into a hero through trials, challenges, and self-discovery. His groundbreaking work, *The Hero with a Thousand Faces*, detailed this journey, breaking it down into several key stages.

Campbell's insights profoundly influenced storytelling in modern movies, books, and pop culture. One of his most famous admirers was George Lucas, who openly credited Campbell's work as the inspiration for the mythology of Star Wars. Lucas structured Luke Skywalker's journey around Campbell's mythical framework, following the classic arc of a reluctant hero who is called to adventure, mentored by a wise figure, tested through great trials, and ultimately transformed by his experiences.

Beyond Star Wars, the hero's journey has shaped countless iconic stories, from *The Lord of the Rings* and *Harry Potter,* to *The Matrix* and *Back to the Future*. Whether set in ancient kingdoms, futuristic galaxies, or magical realms, these stories resonate because they tap into universal themes of courage, self-discovery, and transformation. Campbell's work continues to inspire storytellers, proving that the hero's journey is not just an ancient myth but a timeless reflection of the human experience.

We all have an individual hero's journey to discover, live, and learn from.

When a simplified hero's journey is overlaid onto a cancer journey, it consists of these 7 stages:

1. Life in the Ordinary World- **every day life**

2. Call to Adventure- **a cancer diagnosis**

3. Meeting the Mentor- **working with a team of healthcare professionals**

4. Crossing the Threshold- **stepping into the unknown with treatments**

5. Road of Trials- **overcoming doubts, fears, setbacks, & pain**

6. Seizing the Prize- **defining what life & healing means to you**

7. Return with the Treasure- **remission or lengthening of life with dignity, joy, & inner peace**

Whether that treasure is a full remission and living a long, happy life and then passing away peacefully in our sleep at age 101, or struggling through the pain of cancer with a sense of humor and joy and still passing away, it doesn't really matter. What matters is that we rise to the occasion by becoming the best version of ourselves that we can be, and do our best to live life with no regrets. We are all going to die, so *how we choose* to live is the most important thing.

**I believe that who we become by passing through the refiner's fire of life is the real treasure.**

The 7 Pathways of Healing are designed to be a guide to assist doctors and patients to design an ideal comprehensive treatment plan. They are by no means complete or all-inclusive, because science is learning more about cancer everyday, but they are designed to help you cover all the bases, and make sure your plan doesn't have any major blind spots.

Often, with conventional cancer therapies, the more you do the sicker you feel, while the natural non-invasive approaches outlined in this course are additive, and the more you do, generally the better you will feel, and the greater will be your chances of recovery.

These pathways consist of basically everything else that a medical oncologist does not focus on or have training in. They are just as appropriate for integrative care working with an oncologist as they are for a person using 100% alternative treatments.

I am excited and honored to go through this journey with you. YOU are one of my heroes for choosing to face this challenge, empowered with the knowledge, confidence, and action for your hero's healing journey ahead.

## Chapter 1 Action Steps

Answer either in a journal or a workbook, or discuss with a loved one:

- Where are you on the hero's journey? Which of the 7 stages are you living in now?

- How can you make this experience more enjoyable and channel your inner: Hercules, Luke Skywalker, Princess Leia, Frodo Baggins, Harry Potter, Hermione Granger, or Marty McFly? How can you expand your sense of adventure and humor as you deal with the deep challenges of life?

- Who will be your mentors? Your Obi-Wan Kenobi, Yoda, Merlin, Gandalf, Dumbledore, or Doc Brown?

- What kinds of practitioners do you want to have on your health-care team? (you will probably want to add more to this list as you go down the 7 pathways)

- Who do you want to be on your support team? (special family & friends)

- What resources will you gather to face your Darth Vader, Sauron, Voldemort, or Biff Tannen?

Remember that this is an experiential book, and you will only see results by taking action. So take action on these simple first steps today.

The extra resources at the end of each chapter are in no way required. They are just there as support if you would like to take a deeper dive into the topics of each chapter.

# Resources

**The Hero's Journey: Joseph Campbell on His Life and Work** -Joseph Campbell

**The Power of Myth** - Joseph Campbell & Bill Moyers

**The Writer's Journey - 25th Anniversary Edition: Mythic Structure for Writers**
-Christopher Vogler

# Chapter 2

## Introducing The 7 Pathways of Healing

"The art of healing comes from nature, not from the physician."

-Paracelsus

If you think of The 7 Pathways of Healing as the spokes of a bicycle wheel, you will see the analogy as shown in the diagram.

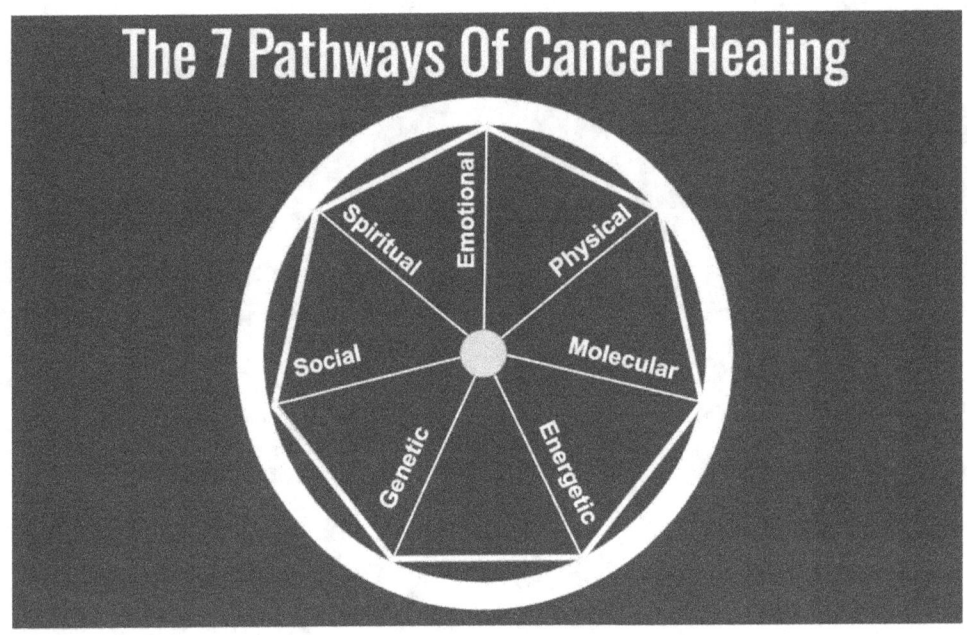

While not all 7 pathways have to be perfectly equal, some attention does need to be given to each one in order to move forward smoothly.

By contrast, only relying on the conventional cancer treatments of chemo, radiation, and surgery is like trying to ride a bike with triangles for wheels, you can't move forward smoothly at all.

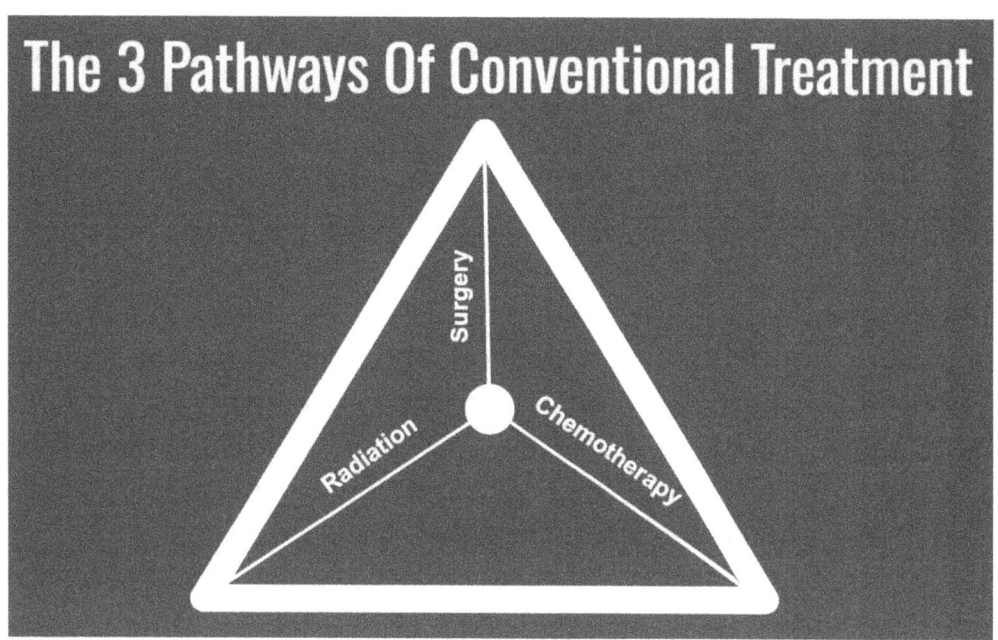

## The 7 Pathways of Healing include:

**The Emotional Pathway-** The emotional pathway deals with the mind-heart-body connection. The mind is part of the body, and the body is part of the mind. In reality, there is no separation between the two. As we will see, emotional traumas can create chronic stress that can be a part of the cause of a cancer diagnosis, and then the diagnosis itself becomes another source of stress that can make emotional burdens even heavier. So the emotional pathway provides tools and resources to balance and heal any negative emotions that may be contributing to poor health, or blocking your healing journey.

**The Physical Pathway-** The physical pathway involves anything to do with touching or moving the physical body. Exercise, massage, deep breathing, and hydrotherapy are examples of physical pathway treatments. Surgery is the main conventional cancer treatment that fits into the physical pathway.

**The Molecular Pathway-** The molecular pathway refers to molecules coming from the outside to the inside of the body through eating or other exposure. This includes foods, herbs, supplements, essential oils, and medications. It also covers the avoidance of toxic and dangerous molecules that can contribute to disease. Chemotherapy is the main conventional treatment that fits into the molecular pathway.

**The Energetic Pathway-** The energetic pathway encompasses therapies that use either measurable energies such as light or electricity, or non-measurable biofield energies such as those used in energy medicine, Reiki, Quantum Touch, or homeopathy. Radiation is the main conventional treatment that fits into the energetic pathway.

**The Genetic Pathway-** The genetic pathway involves understanding our personal genetics and the newer science of epigenetics and how that applies to the cancer process. There are many genes that may become activated in cancer such as BRCA, BCL, p53, MTOR, and RAS. Through optional genetic testing, you can better understand the risks that you and your family have for developing cancer, and then make lifestyle choices to reduce those risks.

**The Social Pathway-** The social pathway is self-explanatory. We are social beings; we need the help, love, touch, and support of our fellow humans to thrive and heal. Many studies have shown dramatically improved cancer outcomes when cancer group therapy or counseling was part of the treatment plan.

**The Spiritual Pathway-** The spiritual pathway is about all of the big questions: Who am I? What is my purpose in life? What is my relationship to Nature, or God, or the Universe? It is also about the main themes taught by many of the world's religions and philosophies including: love, gratitude, compassion, forgiveness, service, etc. There are no right or wrong answers when it comes to healing through the spiritual pathway, but it's critical to do some soul searching and discover your purpose, values, goals, mission, and beliefs about your connection to God, Nature, your Higher Self, and the Universe.

## A Healing Story

Now I want to tell you about a beautiful story that illustrates the power of the 7 pathways of healing. It is found in a 2012 New York Times article called, *The Island Where People Forget To Die* by Dan Buettner.

The article outlines the story of a Greek World War II veteran named Stamatis Moraitis who came to the United States after a war injury and settled on Long Island, New York, then moved to Florida with his family.

33 years later, in 1976, he started feeling short of breath, and after x-rays, his doctor concluded that he had lung cancer, and as he recalls, 9 other doctors confirmed the diagnosis. They gave him 9 months to live. He was in his mid-60s. He thought about staying in America and seeking aggressive cancer treatment at a local hospital, but instead he decided to return home to his Greek island of Ikaria where he could be buried with his ancestors and have a much more affordable funeral.

At first, he spent his days in bed, with his mother and wife tending to him. He reconnected with his faith. On Sunday mornings he would walk up the hill to the tiny Greek Orthodox Chapel where his grandfather once served as a priest. When his childhood friends discovered that he had moved back, they started showing up every afternoon. They'd talk for hours, an activity that often involved a bottle or two of locally produced wine. "I might as well die happy", he thought. In the ensuing months, something strange happened. He says he started to feel stronger. One day, feeling ambitious, he planted some vegetables in the garden. He didn't expect to live to harvest them, but he enjoyed being in the sunshine, breathing the ocean air. He figured his wife could enjoy the fresh vegetables after he was gone. Six months came and went, but he didn't die. Instead he harvested his garden, and feeling emboldened, cleaned up the family vineyard as well.

Gradually easing himself into the island routine, he woke up when he felt like it, worked in the vineyards until the afternoon, made himself lunch, and then took a nap. In the evenings he often walked to the local tavern where he played dominoes past midnight. The years passed. His health continued to improve.

When the article was written in 2012, he was 97 years old according to an official document that he disputes, (he says he's 102), and cancer-free. He never went through chemotherapy, took drugs, or sought therapy of any sort. All he did was move home to Ikaria. The next year, Moriatis died peacefully (and not from cancer) in February, 2013.

This story amazingly encapsulates the 7 Pathways. He moved back home to the Greek island of his youth and lived the lifestyle and ate the diet of his ancestors **(genetic pathway)**. He reconnected with his childhood faith **(spiritual pathway)**. His childhood friends started visiting and hanging out with him **(social pathway)**. He had great support from his wife, mother, and friends **(emotional pathway)**. He started walking, gardening, and re-connecting to the earth in fresh air and sunlight, **(physical and energetic pathways)**. And he ate his own organic vegetables, homemade wine, and wild herbal teas **(molecular pathway)**.

Dan Buettner went on to study the island of Ikaria and many other locations around the world known for their outstanding health and longevity. His findings are compiled into his best-selling book *The Blue Zones*.

This is the power of The 7 Pathways of Healing, if you have been given a few years, or a few months to live, if your doctors have no hope, if you have been told, "there is nothing more we can do for you", or "the treatments have stopped working", there IS still hope for you!

Healing is a matter of changing your life, getting back to your roots, putting your world back into balance, and then letting God, Nature, and your body do the healing.

Of course, most of us can't move to a Greek-island paradise and live a brand new life, but it is an option to consider. It sure would be nice! The purpose of this book is to provide you with the tips, guidance, and framework you need to create your own, "Island Where People Forget to Die" wherever you may live. I know you can do this! Untold thousands have done it before you, and I absolutely know that you can do it too.

## How to Navigate the 7 Pathways

This book will present you with a wide variety of options for each pathway. Don't get overwhelmed or think you have to remember, process, or use all of the information covered. Think of it like a menu at a restaurant. You don't go to a restaurant, read over the whole menu, and then go into a panic because you simply cannot eat or pay for all of the food listed on the entire menu that night. Instead, you thoughtfully look over the menu and order what you want for each course of the meal.

The purpose of this book is to empower you with the information, options, and confidence that you need to assemble a support team, and craft a well-rounded treatment plan that doesn't have any major holes or blind spots in it. I want you to choose at least one of the recommendations for each pathway. I will usually recommend at least 2-3 per pathway, because up to a point, the more of these you do, the healthier you will become.

These treatments generally don't have negative side effects. They have positive side effects that spill over to other areas of life, creating an upward spiral of healing. However, those with extreme or "Type-A" personalities will need to move forward with balance and restraint. Recovery is a marathon not a sprint. You can easily burn yourself out going to so many practitioners, and doing so many home therapies that you have no time to rest, breathe, or actually live your life. So the goal is to walk the middle path and do enough to heal, but not so much that it causes any increased stress, fatigue, or burnout.

Conventional cancer treatments basically have one category for the molecular pathway (chemotherapy), one category for the physical pathway (surgery), and one category for the energetic pathway (radiation). This leaves massive blind spots in the other pathways of healing including the emotional, social, genetic, and spiritual pathways. It also leaves gaping holes, ignoring hundreds of the other cancer-healing treatments that science has uncovered in the molecular, physical, and energetic pathways.

I don't want this to happen to you. Riding a bicycle with triangular wheels is really challenging. I want you to have the knowledge and confidence to cover all of the bases for healing so that you and your loved ones can move forward with no regrets. So that no matter what happens, you can say, "I did my best with all the resources that I had at the time", you can then safely leave the rest to Infinite Grace.

## Chapter 2 Action Steps

Take a few minutes to either journal in a workbook, or discuss with a loved one:

- What are your thoughts and feelings about what this diagnosis of cancer might mean for you and your family?

- Some patients have said that cancer is the best thing that ever happened to them, since it caused them to reassess the direction or the priorities of their life. Pretend that this is true for you. What are the potential 'silver linings' for this experience?

- What might your cancer be trying to teach you? Write a letter from the point of view of your cancer explaining the messages it is trying to teach you. Why might it be trying to get your attention?

- What are some of your goals for the rest of your life?

- Which of the 7 Pathways are the most out of balance in your life right now?

- Which Pathways are you most excited to learn more about?

# Resources

**The Blue Zones**  -Dan Buettner

**The Island Where People Forget To Die**  -Dan Buettner
https://www.nytimes.com/2012/10/28/magazine/the-island-where-people-forget-to-die.html

# Chapter 3

# The 4 Major Goals of Natural Healing: Cleanse, Nourish, Circulate, & Rest

"Each patient carries his own doctor inside him."

-Norman Cousins -Bestselling Author of *Anatomy of an Illness*

### Cleanse

We live in a toxic world with over 80,000 types of industrial chemicals that permeate our water, air, soil, homes, and bodies. While the daily toxic exposures are usually tiny, the cumulative health effects can be massive. Fortunately, the human body has an exceptional detoxification system that works daily to transform and eliminate these harmful molecules from our systems. However, due to lower quality of nutrition and a higher toxic burden in our food, air, and water, modern humans have detox systems that are overwhelmed.

Many health conditions such as cancer, fatigue, obesity, depression, and neurodegenerative disease can all be related to excess toxins trapped in the body. We can all take steps to purify our air, water, food, and homes to reduce the constant inflow of chemicals into our lives. Periodic cleanses are another answer to this challenge.

The body has two main routes of elimination that function like sewer pipes to rid the body of internal and external toxins. These big 2 are the urinary system for liquids and the large intestine for solids. Poisons (either from our own cellular metabolism or from food, air, water, or other pollution) travel through the bloodstream on a daily basis. These poisons are then filtered and processed by the liver in what is known as phase I and phase II detoxification. The liver first transforms the chemical through an intricate series of enzymes known as the cytochrome P450 system (phase I), and then it adds a molecule to the toxin to make it easier for the body to eliminate (phase II). More solid or fat-soluble toxins are transported from the liver into the intestinal system to be eliminated through the bowels. More water-soluble poisons are filtered through the kidneys and then eliminated in the urine.

Secondary routes of toxin elimination include the lungs and skin. For this reason **deep breathing of fresh air, exercise, skin brushing, and sauna therapy** are all recommended detoxification habits. Any poisons not efficiently excreted by the body end up being stored in our fat cells or other tissues.

Other healthy detoxification habits include: **massage, hot/cold contrast showers, enemas, colon hydrotherapy, and increasing the intake of targeted supplements such as psyllium husks, bentonite clay, and apple pectin that bind and absorb toxic molecules.** These routes of elimination can be optimized with specific foods, herbs, supplements, and lifestyle habits.

You can slow down toxic exposures by:

- Choosing organic produce and meats as much as you can afford
- Use high-quality filters for drinking water and showers
- Avoid drinking or eating from plastic bottles or containers when possible
- Avoid microwaving any food with plastic or styrofoam as this will leach synthetic molecules directly into your food.
- Use natural or homemade cleaning products, fragrances, candles, etc. in your home and car.

## Nourish

Every cell in the body has a need for essential nutrients that must be obtained from outside sources. Too many of us are overfed and undernourished. This means too many calories, and not enough nutrients such as essential fatty acids, vitamins, minerals, amino acids, phytonutrients, and enzymes. There are many reasons for this lack of vital nutrients in the food supply including:

- Depleted soils from over-farming and mono-cropping

- Transportation of food from other countries that lose nutrients in transit
- Processing, canning, and freezing of packaged foods
- Non-organic farming produces inferior crops with lower nutrient levels
- Agricultural breeding for size and yield instead of nutritional value
- Un-natural diets and lifestyles for cows, pigs, chickens, and other food animals

We need to eat the best we can, favoring whole foods, organic produce, brightly-colored fruits and vegetables, and home cooking when possible. Essentially everyone should add quality supplements to their healthy diet. The most recommended supplements include: **a natural whole-food multivitamin (capsules or liquid), antioxidants, essential fatty acids, probiotics, and digestive enzymes.** Other healthy ideas include buying a Juicer and using it 3-6 times per week, and/or buying a powerful high-end blender. These machines allow us to take in more concentrated nutrients from fruits and vegetables without all of the chewing involved in eating and digesting the whole foods. Experiment with juice and smoothie recipes online. Learn to experiment and play with flavors, colors, ingredients, and spices. Just enjoy real food!

## Circulate

To be healthy, humans need to circulate oxygen, blood, and lymphatic fluid to keep every cell vital and strong. Circulation is how the first two steps of cleansing and nourishing happen. Each cell is like a miniature body; it creates waste that needs to be expelled and has nutritional needs that have to be fed. Circulation of oxygen from the lungs into the bloodstream feeds every cell with the fuel it needs to create energy for living.

Blood circulates from the heart to the periphery and back once every minute. It carries oxygen attached to red blood cells, as well as amino acids, fats, sugars, vitamins, and minerals to every cell. If any area of the body is ever cut off from the normal supply of blood or lymphatic circulation, the cells in that area begin to starve, and chronic lack of circulation can cause pain, numbness, infections, possible cancer, and tissue destruction.

Lymph is a clear yellowish fluid similar to blood plasma and carries white blood cells and cellular waste from the spaces in between cells into the bloodstream for processing and removal. Because the lymphatic system does not have a central pump like the blood does, it depends on other forces to keep it flowing properly. Deep breathing, any exercise or muscle movement, massage, and bouncing on a large or mini-trampoline can all help move lymph more efficiently. Circulation can be increased by some of the following activities:

- Daily exercise like walking, jogging, swimming, yoga, etc
- Deep belly breathing throughout the day
- Dry skin brushing each morning before a shower. Use light quick strokes with a natural bristle brush from the hands and feet, and brushing inward towards the heart.
- Alternating hot/cool showers each morning. 1 minute hot water, then 30 seconds cool water, repeated 4-6 times. The contrast in temperature drives the blood to the core of the body and then to the surface over and over, creating a powerful pumping action that can feel like the equivalent of a 30-minute workout.
- Body work such as massage, cranial sacral therapy, and chiropractic help keep circulation channels flowing.
- Culinary herbs such as: cayenne pepper, black pepper, jalapenos, ginger, garlic, and horseradish all stimulate blood flow and circulation.

## Rest

Life on earth depends on cycles of day and night, light and dark, activity and rest. Without rest, the human body has no chance to recover, recharge, and heal from the wear and tear of the day. Rest comes in many forms including: night-time sleep, naps, meditation, leisure activities, and vacations. Getting at least 7-9 hours of sleep per night is an ideal that is becoming more rare in modern society. If insomnia or lack of sleep is a problem, work with a Naturopathic Doctor or other holistic professional for help in getting restful sleep. Make sure rest is a priority for you by addressing the following areas:

- Make it a goal to get 7-9 hours of sleep each night

- Learn to take breaks from work or study a few minutes out of every hour
- Practice meditation with silence, guided visualizations, or soothing music
- Take time to explore new and familiar leisure activities and hobbies
- Take regular vacations, and take periodic camping or other getaways that allow you to connect with nature, and unplug from cell phones, electronics, email, and wifi signals for a few days.

## Chapter 3 Action Steps

Take a few minutes to either journal in a workbook, or discuss with a loved one:

- What are the easiest changes you can start to make to optimize your cleanse, nourish, circulate, or rest habits?
- Starting today, what is the lowest hanging fruit for change? Can you order a shower filter or a dry skin brush online?
- Can you throw away some candy or other processed junk food from your kitchen?
- Can you take a walk around the block and breathe deeply?
- Can you turn off your phone 2 hours before bedtime so you are ready for better sleep?

We will cover these habits in more detail in the actual 7 Pathways chapters, but what are the **1 or 2 easiest and most enjoyable changes you can begin today or tomorrow** to build momentum for the road ahead?

# Chapter 4

## Basic Concepts About Cancer

"Cancer is a word, not a sentence."

- John Diamond

First of all, cancer is not a tumor, or a thing, or a disease you catch like a cold. It's a process. It would be more accurate to say that your body is 'cancer-ing' than that you 'have cancer'. I don't think this language will ever really catch on, but this is a useful way to look at it.

This is why cancer often comes back after it's removed or slowed down by surgery, radiation, or chemo, because the visible lump or tumor was removed, but nothing was ever done to change the course of the original cancer *process*.

### The 4 main known root causes of cancer include:

**Radiation**- This comes in 2 varieties. Ionizing radiation like X-rays, CT scans, and Nuclear fallout.

And non-ionizing radiation from: Overexposure to sunlight, Cell phones, Wifi routers, Bluetooth, Power lines, Smart meters, Excessive airline travel, etc.

**Organisms**- Bacteria, Viruses, or Parasites

**Chemicals**- Carcinogens in Tobacco, Alcohol, Air Pollution, Water Pollution, Gasoline, Cleaning Products, Used Motor Oil, Solvents, Heavy Metals, Pesticides, Paints, Cosmetics, Preservatives, Artificial Colors, Artificial Sweeteners, Synthetic Vitamins, Some Pharmaceutical Drugs, and many more categories.

**Emotional or Physical Traumas**- Emotional traumas have often been correlated to a subsequent cancer diagnosis months or years later.

Physical traumas, including surgeries, have been linked to sometimes developing cancer in the area that was traumatized. For example, if a woman is in a car accident and her breast is crushed against the seat belt, then breast cancer will be more likely to develop in that breast with the previous trauma. My sister had gallbladder removal surgery, and then about 2 years later she was diagnosed with an aggressive bile-duct cancer. The doctors believed it could have been related to the surgical trauma from the gallbladder removal in the same area as her bile duct.

The thing that these 4 causes have in common is that they are all chronic irritants that the body has a hard time getting rid of or healing completely, because they are usually constant daily exposures found in our air, water, phones, cigarettes, food, mind, etc. Physical and emotional traumas can trigger chemical cascades inside of the body like: stress hormones, immunosuppressant molecules, growth factors, clotting factors, or fibrin scar tissue. If the body doesn't restore balance after the trauma, these internal chemicals then become chronic irritants that can eventually trigger the cancer process.

This brings us to the next point. Cancer is often referred to as "a wound that doesn't heal". The wounds are usually caused by one or many of the above causes. Then its efforts to heal are constantly thwarted by repeated exposures, just like a scab that is torn off over and over and doesn't ever get a chance to fully heal.

## Health Goals That Are Related To The Cancer Process

These goals will be covered by following the rest of the 7 Pathways Program, so don't worry about the details. This is just background knowledge to build your understanding of the cancer process and some of the terms surrounding it.

**Improve Mitochondrial Health-** As you probably learned in High School Biology, the mitochondria are little organs inside our cells responsible for creating energy at the molecular level. One of the most likely theories of the central cause of cancer is mitochondrial dysfunction. The cell loses the power to create energy normally through the burning of glucose and oxygen as fuel, so it flips into an alternative pathway for creating energy by using fermentation to create energy without oxygen. This process is very inefficient and requires way more glucose to create the same amount of energy.

This is the science behind Positron Emission Tomography (PET) scans for cancer. Radiolabeled glucose is injected into the veins, then the active areas of cancer soak up that glucose like a sponge because they are so hungry for sugar because of their inefficient way of creating energy. By healing and rebuilding our mitochondria we can restore proper cell metabolism, and potentially help cells revert back to the healthier process of using glucose and oxygen for fuel.

**Boost & Educate the Immune System-** The immune system is an intricate network of cells, tissues, and antibodies that work together with incredible harmony throughout the body. Cancer cells seek to block or hide from the immune system. Specialized cells that have an affinity for killing cancer cells include: natural killer cells (aka NK cells) and macrophages which is Greek for "big eaters". These are like blobs that surround cancerous cells, then kill and digest them. There are certain actions you can take in the physical, molecular, and emotional pathways that can increase natural killer cell and macrophage activity, thus increasing your body's ability to take out and clean up cancer cells.

**Block Angiogenesis-** Angiogenesis comes from the Greek words that mean "vessel" & "beginning" so angiogenesis is the medical term for creating new blood vessels in the body. Sometimes angiogenesis is good. If you have a blocked artery to your heart, angiogenesis can create new blood vessels to supply blood to your heart. If you have a severe wound, angiogenesis can form new blood vessels to supply the tissues with blood and nutrients.

However, in the cancer process, a tumor uses angiogenesis to create new blood vessels to supply the tumor with blood and nutrients. So while not all angiogenesis in the body is bad, if you have active cancer you want to do everything you can to block angiogenesis so that it will starve the tumor of the nutrients that it needs to grow and spread. Many of the foods, herbs, and supplements in the molecular pathway have the ability to block or slow down this dangerous process.

**Reduce Oxidative Damage-** Oxidation in metals is called rust, the metal breaks down in response to damaging chemical reactions with oxygen and moisture. Every cell in our body is actually powered by oxidizing glucose or other fuels combined with oxygen to create the adenosine triphosphate or ATP molecules that drive all the functions of life at the cellular level. So oxidation is a good thing because it's what keeps us alive, but too much oxidation causes internal damage similar to rust in a junkyard.

The body is performing a constant balancing act of oxidants versus antioxidants. I'm sure you've heard of antioxidants in foods and supplements like vitamins C, A, E, and Selenium, but just as critical are the internal antioxidants that the body creates such as glutathione (GSH), superoxide dismutase (SOD), and catalase (CAT).

Too much oxidation can cause mutations in DNA and drive the cancer process, so a goal is to balance the oxidative process with enough antioxidants both internal and dietary. Again the molecular pathway is filled with ways to optimize and protect your cells against oxidative damage. If you are working with an oncologist, they will almost always recommend that you not take in any supplemental antioxidants during chemotherapy treatment. While it has never been proven that antioxidants interfere with chemo, it is still best to err on the side of caution and avoid antioxidant supplements during active chemotherapy.

**Lower & Balance Blood Sugar-** Because of metabolic changes in cancer cells they are much more dependent on blood glucose than average cells. Because of this, diets that are high in processed carbohydrates and sugars can increase the cancer process. If you have type 1 or type 2 diabetes, or have a high carbohydrate diet, you will need to work with your healthcare providers and take extra steps to reduce your average blood sugar measured by hemoglobin A1c levels to between 5 - 5.5 if possible. Steps in the physical and molecular pathways can help with this.

**Reduce Inflammation-** Just like angiogenesis or oxidation, inflammation is something that needs to be carefully balanced in the body. If you have a wound or sprain your ankle inflammation is part of the healing process and is necessary and healthy for tissue repair, but chronic inflammation is toxic to the body and can stimulate or worsen the cancer process. Prostaglandins are molecules the body makes out of fats that control inflammation in the body; some prostaglandins are inflammatory and others are anti-inflammatory. Many items in the molecular, energetic, and physical pathways can reduce and balance inflammation throughout the body.

**Balance pH**- Cancer cells thrive in an acidic environment, and they create a more acidic zone around the tumor. This in turn helps the cancer to grow faster and be more invasive. By having the right range of acid/base pH in our tissues, it creates a healthier environment for cancer healing. Simple diet and lifestyle changes can create a more ideal pH balanced state in your tissues.

**Improve Detoxification**- Because toxic chemicals are some of the major root causes of cancer, improving the rate of detoxification of the tissues is a major goal. Detoxification is a holistic process that involves the physical, energetic, molecular, and emotional pathways.

**Prevent Metastasis**- Biopsies and surgery can inadvertently cause a spread of cancer cells to other parts of the body (metastasis). Cancer cells can also do this naturally by secreting enzymes known as matrix metalloproteinases (MMPs) that degrade and dissolve the connective tissue between cells. They can then get into the bloodstream and spread cancerous tumors to other parts of the body. Natural medicine has various molecules that can help prevent or slow the spread of cancer cells to distant locations.

**Increase Apoptosis**- Apoptosis is programmed cell death when a cell senses that it is no longer healthy enough to be viable. All cancer cells should go into a state of apoptosis and die, but they are able to block apoptosis signals to stay alive indefinitely. Through aspects of the energetic, physical, and molecular pathways we are able to increase the rate of apoptosis in the cancerous cells.

**Reduce Stress And Emotional Trauma**- As mentioned earlier, emotional stresses and traumas are one of the four major root causes of the cancer process. By exploring activities in the emotional pathway you can learn to manage the current stress of an active cancer diagnosis as well as process older buried stresses and traumas. While stress is an ongoing challenge in all human lives, the major unresolved traumas and stresses can become a source of chronic disease if not dealt with and healed.

**Lose Weight If Needed-** Obesity is an independent risk factor for many many types of cancer, and will make any cancers that you do have even worse due to the hormonal and inflammatory effects of excess fat tissue in the body.

**Optimize Sleep-** Multiple studies have revealed that night shift workers have higher rates of cancer than regular day shift workers. Disrupted circadian rhythms and sleep cycles cause many systems in the body to go haywire, and these disordered systems can contribute to the cancer process.

**Connect To Nature-** The human body is created to connect with its natural environment. Modern life has literally disconnected us from nature and the earth. Many aspects of the physical, energetic, and molecular pathways involve reconnecting to the earth through exposure to fresh air, sunlight, and physically touching plants, and the earth.

**Optimize Thyroid, Adrenal, and Sex Hormone Levels-** Optimizing hormones should be a part of every responsible treatment plan, but it is especially important for cancer patients. Proper endocrine balance creates an ideal healing environment to have the best chances of a long and healthy life.

**Fill Your Life With Love, Joy, and Purpose-** To love and be loved, to have joy in life, and to feel like you're living your life on purpose, are goals of most all humans, but it is even more critical for those dealing with a life-threatening illness. None of us know how long we will live, and accidents or illness can take us at any time. By following the emotional, social, and spiritual pathways, you can fill your life with love, family, friendship, and connection, which is the most important part of a life worth living.

# Chapter 4 Action Steps

Take a few minutes to either journal in your workbook, or discuss with a loved one:

- The 4 main causes of cancer are: radiation, organisms, chemicals, & traumas. Which ones seem like they could be potential culprits?

- Do you have long term exposure to 1st or 2nd hand smoke?

- Have you had excessive cellphone use over the past 10-30 years?

- Do you have a job or hobby that adds toxic chemicals to your body on a regular basis?

- Have you had a physical or emotional trauma related to the area of your cancer?

- Have you had a diagnosis of viral hepatitis, H. pylori bacteria, dental problems, or other hidden infections?

- Take time to brainstorm how you can begin to minimize or avoid these 4 causes of cancer in your life. Just as when stopping a car, you have to first take your foot off the gas pedal before you can hit the brakes. One of the first important steps in healing from cancer is to slow the input of toxic radiation, organisms, molecules, and traumas into your life.

# Chapter 5

## The Emotional Pathway

"Cancer is not a medical emergency, it's an emotional emergency."

-Unknown

I don't separate the emotional from the mental. Thoughts create feelings, and feelings create thoughts. The brain and the heart work together as different sides of the same coin to help us process our thoughts and feelings. So this is the pathway of both logic and emotion and how they come together in mind/body medicine

The introductory quote is true; cancer is physically slow growing and often takes many years to spread, but the emotional impact and stress of a cancer diagnosis is immediate. This is the first critical piece to work on if you are stressed, worried, or afraid. So let's get into the research on the emotional pathway.

Research into emotional conditions that have been **associated with poor outcomes** in cancer include:

- Depression
- Excessive stress
- Lack of control over care
- Passivity
- Lack of support
- Pessimism
- Stoic acceptance of your fate
- Hopelessness
- Grief
- Trauma
- Lack of meaning
- Fear
- Belief in a Dr's negative prognosis
- Trying too hard to please others

- Isolation
- Loneliness

Conditions that are associated with **positive outcomes** in cancer include:

- Having a fighting spirit
- Denial of the power of the disease
- Optimism
- Purpose
- Passion
- Service
- Gratitude
- Forgiveness
- Future goals
- Humor
- Daily fun
- Being less blindly obedient to doctors
- Being proactive
- Having social support
- Prayer
- Hope
- Healthy anger
- Assertiveness
- Sadness
- Expressing emotions
- Co-decision making with their doctor

"Find a place inside where there's joy, and the joy will burn out the pain."

-Joseph Campbell

Through the science of psychoneuroimmunology, we know that the immune cells that help fight cancer are 'listening' to our emotions. Negative emotions can suppress the immune system, and positive emotions can literally help stimulate increased antibody production.

## The Emotional Pathway Options

**German New Medicine**- In the late 1970's, German doctor Ryke Geerd Hamer, discovered that emotional traumas are often a trigger for the development of cancer. He was working as a busy doctor when he received a sudden shock that his son had just passed away from a terrible accident. A few months later Dr Hammer was diagnosed with testicular cancer. Curious if this new cancer could have been an expression of the grief from the loss of his son, he researched all of his old patient files and discovered that nearly all of them had also had profound emotional traumas, grief, shock, or loss. He developed this concept into what is now called German New Medicine (GNM) or Germanic Healing Knowledge (GHK) and other doctors around the world have picked up the torch from Dr Hamer and have found that by discovering and processing these

emotional traumas and conflicts, it can help the body to heal physically and be part of reversing the cancer process.

Danny Carroll has survived cancer of the lung, testicle, jaw, and skin. He is the author of *Terminal Cancer is a Misdiagnosis,* which is a short introduction to the topic of German New Medicine.

Essentially, the idea is that there is a biological purpose that the body is trying to fulfill through the cancer process; this is called the biological conflict. For example, a woman's breasts are biologically there to feed and nurture her babies. If there is an emotional conflict related to being able to feed, nurture, or be there for a loved one, then her body could trigger a subconscious compensating mechanism by sending more growth energy to her breasts to produce more milk to nurture that loved one. This extra growth energy can eventually lead to rapidly growing cells of the mammary glands, or breast cancer.

If this conflict with the loved one is able to be resolved, then the body no longer needs to feed the cancer process, and the cancer is more likely to reverse itself. This is a fascinating field of mind-body medicine that deserves your open-minded exploration.

**Humor-** We have all heard that "Laughter is the best medicine." What if this is really true? Norman Cousins, in his book, *The Anatomy of An Illness,* described his battle with a crippling health condition using laughter therapy as a main treatment. Cathy Goodman was a cancer survivor featured in the hit documentary, *The Secret.* She explained that one of the things she did was watch very funny movies, "all we would do is just laugh, laugh, laugh". You can tap into this universal healing power of humor for free. You already know what's funny to you, so just add more of it. Whether it's stand up-comedy specials, Youtube cat videos, improv, live shows, movies, sitcoms, classic 3 Stooges, telling your own jokes- it doesn't matter- just laugh. Do everything you can to laugh every day!

**Counseling**- Lawrence Leshan was a pioneer in the use of psychotherapy to support cancer patients, he focused on the positive traits in each person and how he could support the individual to 'sing their own song' and live

life to their fullest individual expression. His theories are put forth in his book, *Cancer As A Turning Point*. He has stated that 20 years after

adopting this approach, about half of his assumed 'terminal' patients were in remission and still alive. Interestingly, Leshan passed away in 2020 at the age of 100, so his counseling work may have been good for his health as well. Counseling is readily available locally or online, and is often covered by insurance.

**Guided Visualization**- Guided visualization has been taught by many experts over the years including the Silva Mind Control Method, Carl Simonton, Dr Bernie Siegel, Dr Joe Dispenza, and Kelly Howell. It simply consists of closing your eyes and listening to a live or recorded practitioner and allowing your mind to experience the healing imagery. The body then responds to the visualizations by synthesizing hormones, neuropeptides, endorphins, and special immune chemicals called cytokines.

Guided visualization is free, and simple to do. Even many children have been taught to imagine their immune cells as a ship from the old video game *Space Invaders* and the cancer cells as little alien craft that they blast away for a few minutes a day. There are many other visualizations that can be useful as well. Just pick any image of cancer disappearing that resonates with your personality, and repeat this image with feeling and conviction for a few minutes a day. The human imagination is one of the most powerful forces on earth, and has created all of civilization as we know it. It can stimulate profound healing forces as well.

**Affirmations**- are ways of focusing on powerful, positive words that gradually change our conscious and subconscious thoughts. When creating an affirmation, use "I AM" statements. For example: "I am happy and healthy", "Every day, I am growing stronger and healthier", or "I am filled with light, love, and inner peace." Look up more affirmations online or write your own. Repeat them throughout the day especially, right after waking and right before bedtime.

**The Subconscious Mind-** In his pioneering book, *The Biology of Belief,* Dr Bruce Lipton discusses 3 powerful ways to affect our subconscious mind that controls 80-90% of our lives. These 3 are: Hypnotherapy, Mindfulness, & Energy Psychology.

1. **Clinical Hypnotherapy-** is simply visualization & suggestions while in a highly relaxed meditative state. You can either meet in person or online with a certified clinical hypnotherapist, purchase audio hypnosis recordings, or create your own self-hypnosis MP3 to listen to each night as you fall asleep.

2. **Meditation-** There are hundreds of styles of meditation including: mindfulness, Transcendental Meditation (TM), recordings, binaural beats, phone apps like Calm and Headspace, and sensory deprivation float tanks. All of these offer very powerful relaxation, and emotional and physical healing.

3. **Energy Psychology-** refers to a newer growing field of using the body, acupuncture points, or movements to rewire the nervous system in various ways. Some types include: EFT (Emotional Freedom Technique) see below, TFT (Thought Field Therapy) TAT- Tapas Acupressure Technique, Psych-K, and EEM (Eden Energy Medicine).

**Emotional Freedom Technique (EFT)-** Founder Gary Craig created this system of tapping certain emotional acupuncture points while focusing on a disturbing emotion to reduce the perception of stress and emotional traumas. This is such a fast and easy technique for making emotional shifts, that I recommend it to everyone. See **emofree.com** or search EFT on Youtube for more information.

**Eye Movement Desensitization & Reprocessing (EMDR)-**This was originally designed to alleviate the distress associated with traumatic memories. Making specific eye movements while focusing on a painful emotion helps the mind interpret and reprocess these emotions in a different way. Since the eyes are the most direct connection to the nervous system, they are a perfect gateway to help reset thoughts and emotions.

**The Emotion Code**- Dr. Bradley Nelson is a chiropractor who has devoted the last few decades of his life to developing a simple process to discover and heal stuck emotions in the body/mind system. You can learn to do this for yourself or your family by reading his book, watching a demo video on Youtube, or you can visit in person or online with a growing number of Emotion Code practitioners across the globe. My wife and I have learned this simple yet powerful technique, and have used it on each other and with our children with great success.

**Journaling**- This can be a great form of solo therapy that provides a safe place for emotional exploration and healing. Some possibilities are:

- Free writing (3-5 pages without thinking or stopping)
- Write a letter to your cancer thanking it for the lessons you have learned from it
- Journaling about a specific emotional trauma from your past
- Journaling about your future dreams, hopes, goals, and desires
- Journaling about someone you need to forgive

To add more emotional power to writing exercises, you can choose to write about negative emotions on regular loose leaf paper and then burn them in a fireplace or fire pit. As you watch the paper go up in smoke, visualize and feel these emotions release from your heart, mind, and body.

**Tuning Fork or Singing Bowl Sound Therapy**- The book, *Human Tuning* by John Bealieu, offers an introduction to the use of sound vibration for physical and emotional healing. Another method of sound healing is taught and practiced by Eileen McKusick as outlined in her books *Tuning the Human Biofield* and *Electric Body, Electric Health*. This is a very sensory vibrational healing method that I have personally experienced, and it has the power to shake loose some of the old traumas, emotions, and tightness from the tissues.

"Music is a way to tap into the innate knowledge that resides deep in our cells. Music can harmonize us with the Divine. It is capable of bridging

heaven with earth, or our human mortal-self with our spiritual immortal-self."

-Donnie Yance -Best-Selling Author & Cancer Clinician

**Music Therapy-** Music has been part of human culture for at least as long as written history, probably vastly longer. As we all know, music has a direct connection to the emotional centers of our brain. Live music has the power to vibrate the cells of our entire bodies. Trained music therapists can help facilitate incredible healing experiences and visualizations based on specifically chosen music. At the very least, you can collect your favorite songs that bring you joy, peace, and relaxation, and listen to them often while breathing deeply and experiencing bliss in the present moment. Some healing centers combine state of the art sound-vibration therapy with light therapy, and music therapy to create an even more immersive transformation.

**Art Therapy-** Art therapy uses art as a way to express emotions, cope with stress, and improve mental health. It can be a helpful way for people with cancer to deal with the many challenges they face, including the diagnosis itself, treatment, and the side effects of treatment.

There are many benefits to art therapy for cancer patients. It can help reduce stress and anxiety, improve mood, help with pain management, and even enhance the immune system. It can also provide a way for patients to express themselves and their feelings in a safe and supportive environment.

If you are interested in art therapy, there are many online resources available to help you find a qualified therapist in your area.

If you cannot afford or find an art therapist near you, you can still gain many of the benefits by doing your own art therapy at home. You can simply use any paper or sketch book that you have, and any pens, markers, colored pencils, or paints to draw or paint your feelings about your cancer: what it looks like, what physical objects represent it, and what colors it has. Then on another sheet of paper draw whatever symbolizes your powerful body, your completely healthy state in full remission, or your mighty immune cells going to work gobbling up old cancer cells. Art therapy can easily be combined with music therapy for an even more sensory experience.

**Frequency Specific Microcurrent**- In her groundbreaking book, *The Resonance Effect*, Dr Carolyn McMakin shares her life's work in discovering, developing and teaching Frequency Specific Microcurrent therapy. These gentle and imperceptible electrical frequencies can help improve mood, heal the brain after injuries, calm the nervous system, soothe PTSD, and much more.

## Chapter 5 Action Steps

Now that you have heard about all of these emotional pathway techniques, notice which ones you are already doing, which ones you have tried in the past, and which ones have stirred up your interest to try soon.

I recommend trying at least 1-3 three of these on a regular basis to process and heal at the emotional level.

- Out of the therapies that are new to you, decide which one you will try out first, and schedule an appointment or block of time to experience it in the next week.

## Timeline Exercise

Create a time and place where you can be undisturbed for 30-60 minutes. Breathe deeply and relax for at least 30 seconds or so. On a sheet of paper or journal, create an emotional timeline of your life from your earliest memories up to the present day.

What major stresses, accidents, illness, griefs, and traumas have you had throughout your life?

Brainstorm all the highs and lows you can think of, and put them in order on a timeline (either vertical or horizontal). Once you have completed this list with everything you can think of, ponder which ones seem like the most impactful events that caused the most stress or trauma and circle or highlight these.

Which ones do you feel like you have fully processed and healed from, and which ones seem like there is unfinished business, or suppressed, ignored, or stuffed-down feelings?

This highlighted priority list will be a guide as you work with these tools to heal and release the layers of your emotional traumas.

## Resources

### Books:

**Terminal Cancer is a Misdiagnosis** -Danny Carroll

**German New Medicine Experiences in Practice: An introduction to the medical discoveries of Dr. Ryke Geerd Hamer**
-Dr. Katherine Willow

**Anatomy of an Illness as Perceived by the Patient: Reflections on Healing and Regeneration** -Norman Cousins

**The Secret** -Rhonda Byrne

**Cancer As a Turning Point: A Handbook for People with Cancer, Their Families, and Health Professionals** -Lawrence LeShan

**Getting Well Again: The Bestselling Classic About the Simontons' Revolutionary Lifesaving Self-Awareness Techniques**
-O. Carl Simonton MD

**Love, Medicine and Miracles: Lessons Learned about Self-Healing from a Surgeon's Experience with Exceptional Patients**
-Bernie Siegel MD

**You Are the Placebo: Making Your Mind Matter** -Dr. Joe Dispenza

**The Biology of Belief** -Dr. Bruce Lipton

**PSYCH-K...The Missing Peace In Your Life!** -Robert M. Williams

**The EFT Manual** -Gary Craig

**The Emotion Code**  -Dr. Bradley Nelson

**Human Tuning** -John Bealieu

**Tuning the Human Biofield**  -Eileen McKusick

**Electric Body, Electric Health** -Eileen McKusick

**The Resonance Effect**  -Dr. Carolyn McMakin

## Video:

**TEDx Talk: My survival story - what I learned from having cancer**
https://www.youtube.com/watch?v=M5QBH3wDrQY

# Chapter 6

## The Energetic Pathway

"If you want to find the secrets of the universe, think in terms of energy, frequency, and vibration."

-Nikola Tesla

**W**hy the Energetic Pathway? Some of the more scientifically-minded skeptics may ask "Why focus on the energetic pathway? We should only be using what's proven with lab tests, double-blind studies, and what we can see under the microscope."

While what we can perceive with the 5 senses is wonderful, it is not the full story of reality. From the birth of quantum physics over 100 years ago, to studies with the advanced particle accelerators such as the Large Hadron Collider of today, scientists at the cutting edge have learned that particles are not really particles, and that solid matter is not really solid.

If you look at your hand with the most advanced instruments known, and keep zooming in, you will see tissues, then cells, then molecules, then atoms, then protons, neutrons, and electrons, then quarks and other sub-atomic particles, then dancing and vibrating strings of pure energy; at least, according to string theory...

We actually have no idea what things are like at that level, but we do know that there are no solid tangible objects at this level. The most brilliant scientists on the planet have basically come to the conclusion that we, and everything else in the universe, are made of pure vibrating energy.

And that, of course, brings us to what Master Yoda said in *The Empire Strikes Back*,

                **"Luminous beings are we, not this crude matter."**

So while we may consciously live in a physical world that can be measured by the 5 senses, these senses are based on illusions created by our nervous systems. There is no solid matter. When you touch a tabletop, it is energy bouncing off of energy.

So while there may be fewer double-blind human studies proving the effectiveness of some of the energetic pathway treatments, I believe that they are more grounded in reality than most of the other more conventional approaches to improving human health.

## Toxic Energies To Avoid

As mentioned in chapter 4, toxic radiation is one of the four main causes of cancer. Science has proven without question the dangers of ionizing radiation like: nuclear fallout from reactor meltdowns like Chernobyl or Fukushima, x-rays, and CT scans. Non-ionizing radiation includes things like cell phones, Wi-Fi routers, Bluetooth devices, high-tension power lines, microwave ovens, Sunlight, and tanning beds. These sources of electromagnetic radiation also provide a source of chronic irritation to the system that can eventually lead to cancer.

I believe all of these things in excess can contribute to the cancer process. Just as cigarettes were once prescribed and recommended by doctors as being healthy, the evidence has come out that the tobacco companies knew for decades that smoking contributes to cancer.

The major telecommunications companies of today have taken a page out of the playbook of the tobacco companies of 70 years ago. They have hired insider scientists to do fraudulent research that takes the focus off of the numerous studies that prove that cell-phone and other radiation can cause cancer.

The science and politics of cell-phone, Wi-Fi, and Bluetooth radiation are outlined well in books like *Disconnect* by Dr. Devra Davis, and *EMF*d* by Dr Joseph Mercola.

**Steps you can take to avoid toxic energies in your life include:**

- Keep your cell phone on airplane mode whenever not in use.
- Power off your cell phone completely at night before you go to sleep
- Unplug your Wi-Fi router at night, or hardwire your home with ethernet connections that are faster and more secure than Wi-Fi.
- Avoid the use of Bluetooth speakers, earbuds, or other devices.

- Avoid the fad of the 'Smart Home' and keep your home as 'dumb' as possible

- Agree to X-rays and CT scans only when medically necessary

- Get moderate natural sunlight, but avoid sunburns as much as humanly possible.

- Minimize your use of microwave ovens and never stand within 6 ft of a microwave when it is running.

The EMF issue is a deep rabbit hole that can take a long time to sort out, so just use common sense, and do your best to reduce these more harmful energies in your life & home.

## Healing Energy Therapies

**Homeopathy-** Is a complete system of energy medicine that has been practiced all around the world for over 200 years. Based on the principle that "like cures like", a practitioner will match a specific remedy to each patient's complete current mind/body state and pattern of symptoms.

Homeopathy has been used as an adjunctive treatment to reduce the side-effects of conventional cancer treatments, and it has also been used as part of a purely natural treatment program, especially by doctors in India where homeopathy is more mainstream. Doctors Banerji, Ramakrishnan, and Grimmer are the 3 that I am aware of that have worked with and written the most about cancer and homeopathy in the past century. See information about their books in the resource section at the end of the chapter.

**Homeopathic Glandulars-** Often the glands in chronic disease are not working properly. These potentized remedies contain a more optimal energetic blueprint for the glands to resonate with. Glandular remedies include: thyroid, thymus, spleen, gallbladder, pancreas, etc.

**Homeopathic UNDA Compounds-** Sometimes referred to as Biotherapeutic Drainage, each of these liquid remedies is a symphony of remedies in itself. Each remedy is identified by a number and corresponds with a specific organ system or function of the body that can be improved. The remedies are often prescribed as a set of three different numbers; one for the organ system that you are trying to balance, one for the condition or imbalance, and one for the draining or detoxifying of the system. You can search online for "Biotherapeutic Drainage" in your area to find a naturopathic doctor or homeopath trained in this form of medicine to help you select the ideal remedies for your situation.

**Energy Medicine**- Methods of using the biofield of the body to transmit healing energy to the client include: Reiki, Quantum Touch, Eden Energy Medicine, The Bengston Energy Healing Method, and many others.

As a younger man, I was very skeptical of 'energy healing' and I thought it was all a scam. However, in my early 20's, through martial arts training, I was able to learn how to sense this invisible form of energy that is known by different names around the world including: chi, ki, prana, mana, the aura, or the biofield. This opened up a whole new world of unseen healing possibilities for the rest of my life.

William Bengston PhD is the person that I believe has done the most rigorous scientific studies on healing cancer in mice using energy medicine. It is completely harmless and non-invasive, and may have fantastic benefits, so I recommend that everyone try at least 1-3 energy medicine sessions with a professional to see how they enjoy it.

**Hyperthermia**- Is the use of heat to increase the body temperature to up to 108 degrees for a short time. General hyperthermia through saunas helps improve circulation, detoxification, and healing. Regular saunas cause whole-body heating and can be done for only short periods of time, but the portable tent-type saunas allow the head to be out of the heat so you can breathe normal room temperature air allowing the rest of the body to be at higher temperatures for much longer.

Because cancer cells are more fragile than normal cells, hyperthermia can help other cancer treatments, such as chemo and radiation work even better by pre-weakening the cancer cells and making them more susceptible to these conventional treatments. Hyperthermia that is applied locally by a probe is also called thermal ablation.

**Modulated Electrohyperthermia**- The Oncotherm EHY 2000+ is an FDA approved medical device. It uses tissue selectivity with a vibration of 13.56 MHz electrical frequency to create local heating.

Cancer cells are more sensitive to this frequency and heat and are then weakened and destroyed. It also sensitizes cancer cells to help radiation, chemo, or photodynamic therapy to work better as well.

**Photodynamic Therapy (PDT)**- Is the process of ingesting or injecting a photosensitizing molecule, then a few days later, special light treatments cause a burst of oxidation that helps kill the cancer cells. Often near Infra-red light is used to activate the photosensitizing molecule. PDT has been shown to work better when used in combination with Modulated Electrohyperthermia.

**Ultraviolet Blood Irradiation Therapy**- This therapy was popular in the 1940s and 50s as a treatment for sepsis and other serious infections. There are now many different kinds of blood irradiation therapy. Some forms extract blood from a vein, expose it to ultraviolet light, and then return the blood back into the vein as an IV drip.

Through still not fully known mechanisms, this process stimulates the immune system and activates white blood cells to kill infections and cancer cells more effectively. More advanced modern versions of this use an IV catheter that shines laser light directly into the bloodstream of the patient as it is flowing through the veins.

**High-Intensity Focused Ultrasound (HIFU)** - Is a procedure most often used in prostate cancer, but can also be used for pancreatic, breast, prostate, and liver cancers. It uses high-powered sound waves to target and destroy the tumor. It is minimally invasive and considered safer than radiation or surgery. It is guided either by an MRI or an imaging ultrasound. Ask your doctor if this newer treatment makes sense for your type of cancer.

**Bio-Meridian Scanning**- This is also known as electro dermal screening, and is the process of using a machine with probes that helps read whether certain acupuncture points are in or out of balance. This can provide valuable clues to organ systems that need attention, and various foods or substances that should be avoided.

**Acupuncture**- Is the ancient Chinese art of treating various points on the body with micro-thin needles. The specific points treated are based on assessments of the tongue, pulse, reported symptoms, and other body patterns. Acupuncture has been most studied to help with the side effects of chemotherapy and radiation including: nausea, vomiting, pain, immune suppression, and fatigue. Finding an acupuncturist is usually very easy these days through a Google search or Yelp reviews.

**Pulsed Electromagnetic Field Therapy (PEMF)**- This treatment has been shown to have a wide range of benefits for the human body. PEMF can support cancer treatments by enhancing the effectiveness of chemo and radiation therapy, reducing inflammation and pain, and stimulating the immune system.

PEMF works by applying low-frequency electromagnetic fields to the body, which can improve blood circulation, enhance cellular metabolism, and help repair damaged tissues. PEMF can also help with reducing stress and anxiety, improving sleep quality, and promoting overall wellness. By using PEMF therapy in conjunction with traditional cancer treatments, patients usually experience better outcomes, reduced side effects, and an improved quality of life.

The Schumann Resonance is a naturally occurring, extremely low-frequency electromagnetic resonance that exists between the Earth's surface and the atmosphere. It is usually described as vibrating at 7.83 cycles per second. PEMF devices can help mimic this slow steady natural healing vibration of the earth.

**Magnet Therapy**- Static or fixed magnet therapy is a form of medicine that involves the application of magnets to the body to alleviate pain and other health conditions. Magnet therapy has been used to manage various types of pain, including back pain, joint pain, and headaches.

There is some evidence to suggest that it may be beneficial for managing cancer-related pain and the cancer process. Magnet stickers are available online that you can stick like a circular band aid around the area of your cancer or any other area of pain. Magnetic mattress covers are also available so you can sleep in a healing magnetic field for one third of your life.

**Frequency Generators**- are based on the concept that resonant frequencies can shatter specific bacteria, viruses, and different cell types, like an opera singer shattering a crystal glass. Some of these types of devices can be in the $ 10,000 range. The Spooky2 is the most affordable healing frequency generator that I know of.

For less than $350 you can purchase a starter kit and download the software for free. It comes with a library of over 20,000 preset frequency programs for nearly every health condition you can imagine.

## Chapter 6 Action Steps

If you need more convincing about the dangers of radiation from technology, read or listen to 2 or 3 of the books found in the resource section of this chapter including:

- Disconnect -**Dr. Devra Davis**
- EMF*d -**Dr. Joseph Mercola**
- The Invisible Rainbow -**Arthur Firstenberg**
- The Non-Tinfoil Guide to EMFs -**Nicolas Pineault**


- Take some first steps to reduce your exposure to these stressful frequencies. Doing this can reduce headaches, chronic pain, fatigue, improve sleep quality, and potentially decrease the cancer process.

- After reviewing these energetic pathway techniques, notice which ones you are already doing, which ones you have tried in the past, and which ones you would like to schedule soon. I recommend trying at least 1 or 2 of these on a regular basis to continue healing at the energetic level.

- Many, such as homeopathy, acupuncture, photodynamic therapy, and energy medicine, need to be performed by trained individuals. Others, like the Spooky2 frequency generator, are just a one-time purchase and then you can do home treatments without any additional investment.

- Put on your calendar when you will schedule your next energy pathway treatment or purchase a new healing device.

# Resources

## Books:

**Disconnect** -Dr. Devra Davis

**EMF*d** -Dr Joseph Mercola

**The Invisible Rainbow** -Arthur Firstenberg

**The Non-Tinfoil Guide to EMFs** -Nicolas Pineault

**The Banerji Protocols - A New Method of Treatment with Homeopathic Medicines** -Prasanta Banerji

**Cancer: My Homeopathic Method** -Dr. AU Ramakrishnan

**Homeopathy and Cancer, the Philosophy and Clinical Experiences of A. H. Grimmer, M.D.** -A. H. Grimmer & Robin Murphy

**Quantum-Touch: The Power to Heal** -Richard Gordon

**Reiki Healing for Beginners** -David Filipe

**The Energy Cure** -William Bengston

**The Original Reiki Handbook of Dr. Mikao Usui** -Mikao Usui & Christine M. Grimm

## Websites:

https://homeopathycenter.org/new-find-a-homeopath/

https://bengstonresearch.com/

https://www.spooky2.com/

# Chapter 7

## The Molecular Pathway: Part 1- Food

"What most people don't realize is that food isn't just calories; it's information. It actually contains messages that connect to every cell in the body."

- Dr. Mark Hyman

I love food, and eating can be one of the most comforting, nourishing, and satisfying experiences of our lives. However, in modern society we've become disconnected from what 'food' even means. There are as many styles of eating as there are people on this planet so it can be utterly confusing to know what to eat to be healthy. Each body also has different genetic and lifestyle factors that create unique nutritional needs. If you need more support in this area, seek out a qualified naturopathic doctor, nutritionist, or nutritional health coach to help you customize your eating plan to meet your body's specific needs.

There are a few basic principles that we want to keep in mind when thinking about eating for beating cancer. Most of these we have already touched on briefly in previous sections, but we'll review them again here.

- Minimize toxic chemicals, preservatives, pesticides, herbicides, artificial colors & flavors, and artificial sweeteners.

- Maximize whole real foods. 99% of your diet should be foods that only have one ingredient on the label or no label at all. For example: a fish, spinach, a nut, an avocado, an olive, etc.

- Increase brightly-colored plant foods to flood your body with rich flavonoids, polyphenols, terpenes, and other turbocharged natural food molecules.

- Reduce or eliminate sugars and simple or processed carbohydrates to keep blood sugar levels balanced. Proteins and fats are essential for life, but there are no 'essential carbohydrates'.

That said, this chapter will cover how I would strive to eat if I were diagnosed with cancer.

## A Reduced-Calorie Whole-Food Dietary-Confusion Eating Plan

Emphasize rainbow-colored vegetables, fish, and healthy fats. Reduce sugars and grains to as close to zero as possible. Sugar is the primary fuel for cancer, so converting to a ketogenic diet can help starve the cancer cells while still nourishing the healthy cells with ketones.

Normal human metabolism burns glucose to make the high-energy molecules called ATP. Ketones are an alternate fuel source that your cells can switch to when no glucose is around. Your body is brilliant and doesn't want to starve, so you also have pathways to break down proteins and convert those into glucose. So a ketogenic diet means very, very low carbohydrates, just enough protein, and high healthy fats.

I believe that an ideal eating plan for cancer would cycle between a reduced-calorie whole-food ketogenic diet, and a more balanced whole-food diet that includes whole grains like brown rice, barley, rye, quinoa, and buckwheat, sweet potatoes, and richly-pigmented fruits (blueberries, blackberries, raspberries, strawberries, black grapes, cherries, mangosteen, acai, etc) interspersed with short periods of fasting with water and herbal teas only before chemo or radiation treatments, or once or twice a month if not undergoing active treatments. Fasting will be discussed further in The Physical Pathway Chapter.

The rationale for this back and forth cycling between a ketogenic diet and a more moderate-carbohydrate whole-food diet is that the ketogenic diet helps starve cancer cells of the glucose they desperately need to flourish and grow, but cancer cells are still living and intelligent, so they can eventually adapt to a ketogenic diet and start to thrive again. There is an exercise system called P90X that was popular in the early 2000's with workout videos that utilize something called 'muscle confusion'. This just means doing a variety of exercises at different angles and speeds and weights so your muscles don't adapt to any specific movement or exercise. The concept is similar to this eating plan. The idea is to alternate back and forth between a low-calorie ketogenic diet, and a more moderate-carbohydrate Mediterranean style diet that's filled with whole foods that have anti-cancer properties like sweet potatoes, grapes, and berries.

Cancer cells are more fragile and have a harder time shifting gears between these fuels of glucose and ketones, so they can become even more weakened and struggle to adapt when using this 'dietary confusion' method.

## What To Eat for the Ketogenic Phase

**Vegetables** (avoid high-carb vegetables like: white potatoes, sweet potatoes, beets, and carrots) Focus on the color green (Spinach, Kale, Broccoli, Brussels sprouts, Chard, Mustard Greens, Peppers, Cucumbers, Zucchini, Celery, Parsley, Cilantro, etc, etc.), and sea vegetables (kelp, dulse, wakame, bladderwrack). All other bright naturally-colored or white vegetables are great too (radish, yellow squash, bell peppers, garlic, onions, cauliflower, cabbage, etc) Open up your eyes to see the rainbow of colors available when shopping in the produce section.

**Mushrooms-** White Button Mushrooms, Cremini, Portobello, Shiitake, Maitake, Oyster, Porcini, etc

**Fish-** Albacore Tuna, Wild Salmon, Herring, Anchovies, Sardines, Mackerel, Trout, Pollock.

**Meat-** Small amounts of organic free-range chicken, turkey, deer, or other wild game.

**Healthy Fats-** Avocados, Olives, Nuts, Seeds, Coconut Milk, Coconut Oil, Organic Butter, Avocado Oil, Olive Oil, Cold-pressed Flax Oil

**All Culinary Herbs and Seasonings-** including: garlic, onion, ginger, turmeric, lemon juice, lime juice, italian seasonings, pepper, chili powder, basil, sage, oregano, Montreal steak seasoning, etc

**Sweeteners-** Small amounts of Stevia, Xylitol, or Monk Fruit extracts

**Bone broth & Vegetable Broth-** For drinks and soup bases.

Build most of your calories around the healthy fats: olives, avocados, coconuts, and nuts as much as possible. These can be served on beds of cooked or raw greens, salads, or veggie stir frys.

**Beverages-** purified filtered water, herbal teas

**Alcohol-** If you do choose to drink alcohol, it must be limited to one serving per day for women, or 2 servings per day for men, or less (because of the different way genders metabolize alcohol). Try to keep it to the occasional glass of red wine since it has more cancer-fighting polyphenols. More consumption than this has been linked to increased risk for many types of cancers.

## What to Avoid

Grains and Flours, Sugars, Artificial Sweeteners, Processed Meats, Fruit, Dairy, Unhealthy fats (hydrogenated oils, shortening, margarine, trans fats, canola oil, soybean oil, 'vegetable' oil) Any Processed or Packaged Foods.

This phase can be anywhere from 2 to 3 weeks out of each month depending on your mood, or how much you enjoy the super-low-carb eating plan.

Then for the other 1-2 weeks of the month you would eat all of the same foods on the keto plan with the addition of:

**Whole grains-** like brown rice, barley, rye, quinoa, and buckwheat

**Legumes-** all types of beans and lentils

**Sweeter vegetables-** like Sweet potatoes, carrots, and beets

**Richly-pigmented fruits-** blueberries, blackberries, raspberries, strawberries, black grapes, cherries, mangosteen, acai, etc

**I am not a fan of corn, wheat, or soy** for this phase because of the problematic genetic modification, spraying of chemicals, depleted soils, etc on these 3 mega crops.

## Specific Foods With Anticancer Properties

Here are some of the foods that have scientific research for their anticancer properties that are available at most local grocery stores. They are listed in alphabetical order.

**Aloe (Aloe vera)-** Studies on aloe vera have shown potential anti-cancer properties attributed to its active compounds. Research indicates that aloe vera exhibits anti-inflammatory, antioxidant, and immune-modulating effects, which can impede cancer cell growth. Additionally, some studies suggest that aloe vera components could inhibit tumor formation and induce cancer cell death in certain types of cancer. In addition to direct anti-cancer properties, it is also a powerful topical first aid for radiation burns on the skin of treated areas. Aloe vera juice is readily available in most grocery and other health food stores.

Majumder R, Das CK, Mandal M. Lead bioactive compounds of Aloe vera as potential anticancer agent. Pharmacol Res. 2019 Oct;148:104416. doi: 10.1016/j.phrs.2019.104416. Epub 2019 Aug 27. PMID: 31470079.

Sánchez M, González-Burgos E, Iglesias I, Gómez-Serranillos MP. Pharmacological Update Properties of *Aloe Vera* and its Major Active Constituents. Molecules. 2020 Mar 13;25(6):1324. doi: 10.3390/molecules25061324. PMID: 32183224; PMCID: PMC7144722.

Tungkasamit T, Chakrabandhu S, Samakgarn V, Kunawongkrit N, Jirawatwarakul N, Chumachote A, Chitapanarux I. Reduction in severity of radiation-induced dermatitis in head and neck cancer patients treated with topical aloe vera gel: A randomized multicenter double-blind placebo-controlled trial. Eur J Oncol Nurs. 2022 Aug;59:102164. doi: 10.1016/j.ejon.2022.102164. Epub 2022 Jun 17. PMID: 35767935.

**Beets (Beta vulgaris)**- Beet root and leaf extracts have been shown to induce apoptosis and decrease cell proliferation, angiogenesis, and inflammation in cervical, skin, liver, lung, and esophageal cancers. Beets contain molecules such as betaine, betanin, lycopene, β-carotene, and lutein that have all shown anti-cancer activity. It has been studied as a chemopreventive that helps with normalizing inappropriate gene activities in cancer cells.

Romero SA, Pavan ICB, Morelli AP, Mancini MCS, da Silva LGS, Fagundes I, Silva CHR, Ponte LGS, Rostagno MA, Bezerra RMN, Simabuco FM. Anticancer effects of root and beet leaf extracts (Beta vulgaris L.) in cervical cancer cells (HeLa). Phytother Res. 2021 Nov;35(11):6191-6203. doi: 10.1002/ptr.7255. Epub 2021 Sep 8. PMID: 34494317.

Ninfali P, Antonini E, Frati A, Scarpa ES. C-Glycosyl Flavonoids from Beta vulgaris Cicla and Betalains from Beta vulgaris rubra: Antioxidant, Anticancer and Antiinflammatory Activities-A Review. Phytother Res. 2017 Jun;31(6):871-884. doi: 10.1002/ptr.5819. Epub 2017 May 2. PMID: 28464411.

**Black Pepper (Piper nigrum)**- Some of black pepper's medicinal molecules include: piperine, kusunokinin, and piperlongumine. The latter compound has been studied to selectively kill cancer cells, and also increases the cancer-killing ability of the chemo drug cisplatin. Essential oils from black pepper were shown to have anti-tumor effects in triple negative breast cancer. This common spice is often added to herbal formulas to enhance their absorption and effectiveness.

Sriwiriyajan S, Sukpondma Y, Srisawat T, Madla S, Graidist P. (-)-Kusunokinin and piperloguminine from Piper nigrum: An alternative option to treat breast cancer. Biomed Pharmacother. 2017 Aug;92:732-743. doi: 10.1016/j.biopha.2017.05.130. Epub 2017 Jun 4. PMID: 28586745.

Roh JL, Kim EH, Park JY, Kim JW, Kwon M, Lee BH. Piperlongumine selectively kills cancer cells and increases cisplatin antitumor activity in head and neck cancer. Oncotarget. 2014 Oct 15;5(19):9227-38. doi: 10.18632/oncotarget.2402. PMID: 25193861; PMCID: PMC4253430.

Zhang M, Qiu B, Sun M, Wang Y, Wei M, Gong Y, Yan M. Preparation of Black pepper (Piper nigrum L.) essential oil nanoparticles and its antitumor activity on triple negative breast cancer in vitro. J Food Biochem. 2022 Dec;46(12):e14406. doi: 10.1111/jfbc.14406. Epub 2022 Sep 19. PMID: 36121189.

**Black Walnut (Juglans nigra)**- Walnuts, walnut husks, and walnut leaves all have varying anti-cancer properties. Among many other things, they contain ellagic acid, juglone, linoleic acid, and oleic acid. They have been studied for effects against colon, renal, esophageal, and many other cancers.

Hardman WE. Walnuts have potential for cancer prevention and treatment in mice. J Nutr. 2014 Apr;144(4 Suppl):555S-560S. doi: 10.3945/jn.113.188466. Epub 2014 Feb 5. PMID: 24500939; PMCID: PMC3952627.

Carvalho M, Ferreira PJ, Mendes VS, Silva R, Pereira JA, Jerónimo C, Silva BM. Human cancer cell antiproliferative and antioxidant activities of Juglans regia L. Food Chem Toxicol. 2010 Jan;48(1):441-7. doi: 10.1016/j.fct.2009.10.043. Epub 2009 Oct 31. PMID: 19883717.

Catanzaro E, Greco G, Potenza L, Calcabrini C, Fimognari C. Natural Products to Fight Cancer: A Focus on *Juglans regia*. Toxins (Basel). 2018 Nov 14;10(11):469. doi: 10.3390/toxins10110469. PMID: 30441778; PMCID: PMC6266065.

**Blueberry (Vaccinium cyanococcus)**- Blueberries contain molecules that have anti-inflammatory, anti-obesity, anti-cancer, neuroprotective, antioxidant, and other healthy actions. Pterostilbene is one of the primary antioxidant components of blueberries, and it has been shown to inhibit cancer growth, trigger apoptosis, and slow metastasis.

McCormack D, McFadden D. Pterostilbene and cancer: current review. J Surg Res. 2012 Apr;173(2):e53-61. doi: 10.1016/j.jss.2011.09.054. Epub 2011 Oct 21. PMID: 22099605.

Chen RJ, Kuo HC, Cheng LH, Lee YH, Chang WT, Wang BJ, Wang YJ, Cheng HC. Apoptotic and Nonapoptotic Activities of Pterostilbene against Cancer. Int J Mol Sci. 2018 Jan 18;19(1):287. doi: 10.3390/ijms19010287. PMID: 29346311; PMCID: PMC5796233.

Baby B, Antony P, Vijayan R. Antioxidant and anticancer properties of berries. Crit Rev Food Sci Nutr. 2018;58(15):2491-2507. doi: 10.1080/10408398.2017.1329198. Epub 2017 Aug 14. PMID: 28609132.

**Cabbage (Brassica oleracea)**- Research has revealed anti-cancer mechanisms linked to its bioactive compounds such as: glucosinolates, which are metabolized into bioactive compounds like sulforaphane and indole-3-carbinol. These compounds have shown the ability to induce detoxification enzymes, which may help neutralize carcinogens and reduce cancer risk. Additionally, Brassica family vegetables possess antioxidant and anti-inflammatory effects, reducing oxidative stress and chronic inflammation, known contributors to cancer development. Furthermore, these vegetables have been associated with inhibiting the proliferation of cancer cells and influencing certain signaling pathways crucial for tumor growth.

Nazeri M, Nemati H, Khazaei M. Nrf2 antioxidant pathway and apoptosis induction and inhibition of NF-κB-mediated inflammatory response in human prostate cancer PC3 cells by Brassica oleracea var. acephala: An in vitro study. Mol Biol Rep. 2022 Aug;49(8):7251-7261. doi: 10.1007/s11033-022-07507-w. Epub 2022 May 26. PMID: 35614167.

Cuellar-Nuñez ML, Luzardo-Ocampo I, Lee-Martínez S, Larrauri-Rodríguez M, Zaldívar-Lelo de Larrea G, Pérez-Serrano RM, Camacho-Calderón N. Isothiocyanate-Rich Extracts from Cauliflower (*Brassica oleracea* Var. Botrytis) and Radish (*Raphanus sativus*) Inhibited Metabolic Activity and Induced ROS in Selected Human HCT116 and HT-29 Colorectal Cancer Cells. Int J Environ Res Public Health. 2022 Nov 13;19(22):14919. doi: 10.3390/ijerph192214919. PMID: 36429638; PMCID: PMC9691161.

Smiechowska A, Bartoszek A, Namieśnik J. Przeciwrakotwórcze właściwości glukozynolanówzawartych w kapuście (Brassica oleracea var. capitata) oraz produktów ich rozpadu [Cancer chemopreventive agents: glucosinolates and their decomposition products in white cabbage (Brassica oleracea var. capitata)]. Postepy Hig Med Dosw (Online). 2008 Apr 2;62:125-40. Polish. PMID: 18388852.

**Cinnamon (Cinnamomum verum & zeylanicum)** - This common spice is a powerhouse of medicinal value that can help increase circulation, lower average blood sugar, and has anti-inflammatory effects. It has many molecules that have been studied including cinnamaldehyde, cinnamic acid, and polyphenols. It has shown anti-cancer effects including the ability to trigger apoptosis and cancer cells and reduce angiogenesis.

Perng DS, Tsai YH, Cherng J, Kuo CW, Shiao CC, Cherng JM. Discovery of a novel anti-cancer agent targeting both topoisomerase I and II in hepatocellular carcinoma Hep 3B cells in vitro and in vivo: Cinnamomum verum component 2-methoxycinnamaldehyde. J Drug Target. 2016 Aug;24(7):624-34. doi: 10.3109/1061186X.2015.1132221. Epub 2016 Jan 21. PMID: 26707867.

Aggarwal S, Bhadana K, Singh B, Rawat M, Mohammad T, Al-Keridis LA, Alshammari N, Hassan MI, Das SN. *Cinnamomum zeylanicum* Extract and its Bioactive Component Cinnamaldehyde Show Anti-Tumor Effects *via* Inhibition of Multiple Cellular Pathways. Front Pharmacol. 2022 Jun 2;13:918479. doi: 10.3389/fphar.2022.918479. PMID: 35774603; PMCID: PMC9237655.

**Cranberry (Vaccinium macrocarpon)**- This grocery store gem has known anticancer and cancer-preventative molecules including flavonols, proanthocyanidins, and anthocyanins. Along with its known antioxidant effects, it has been shown to inhibit the matrix metalloproteinase enzymes that contribute to metastasis.

Ankola AV, Kumar V, Thakur S, Singhal R, Smitha T, Sankeshwari R. Anticancer and antiproliferative efficacy of a standardized extract of *Vaccinium macrocarpon* on the highly differentiating oral cancer KB cell line athwart the cytotoxicity evaluation of the same on the normal fibroblast L929 cell line. J Oral Maxillofac Pathol. 2020 May-Aug;24(2):258-265. doi: 10.4103/jomfp.JOMFP_129_20. Epub 2020 Sep 9. PMID: 33456234; PMCID: PMC7802834.

Déziel B, MacPhee J, Patel K, Catalli A, Kulka M, Neto C, Gottschall-Pass K, Hurta R. American cranberry (Vaccinium macrocarpon) extract affects human prostate cancer cell growth via cell cycle arrest by modulating expression of cell cycle regulators. Food Funct. 2012 May;3(5):556-64. doi: 10.1039/c2fo10145a. Epub 2012 Mar 5. PMID: 22388548.

Déziel BA, Patel K, Neto C, Gottschall-Pass K, Hurta RA. Proanthocyanidins from the American Cranberry (Vaccinium macrocarpon) inhibit matrix metalloproteinase-2 and matrix metalloproteinase-9 activity in human prostate cancer cells via alterations in multiple cellular signaling pathways. J Cell Biochem. 2010 Oct 15;111(3):742-54. doi: 10.1002/jcb.22761. PMID: 20626034.

**Dill (Anethum graveolens)**- This famous pickle spice has many medicinal qualities including the reduction of gas, reducing stomach pain, and improving bad breath. It has also been found to trigger apoptosis in many cancer cell types.

Al-Oqail MM, Farshori NN. Antioxidant and Anticancer Efficacies of *Anethum graveolens* against Human Breast Carcinoma Cells through Oxidative Stress and Caspase Dependency. Biomed Res Int. 2021 May 4;2021:5535570. doi: 10.1155/2021/5535570. PMID: 33997002; PMCID: PMC8112917.

Mohammed FA, Elkady AI, Syed FQ, Mirza MB, Hakeem KR, Alkarim S. Anethum graveolens (dill) - A medicinal herb induces apoptosis and cell cycle arrest in HepG2 cell line. J Ethnopharmacol. 2018 Jun 12;219:15-22. doi: 10.1016/j.jep.2018.03.008. Epub 2018 Mar 9. PMID: 29530611.

Tavakkol Afshari HS, Homayouni Tabrizi M, Ardalan T, Jalili Anoushirvani N, Mahdizadeh R. *Anethum Graveolens* Essential Oil Nanoemulsions (AGEO-NE) as an Exclusive Apoptotic Inducer in Human Lung Adenocarcinoma (A549) Cells. Nutr Cancer. 2022;74(4):1411-1419. doi: 10.1080/01635581.2021.1952450. Epub 2021 Jul 20. PMID: 34282978.

**Figs (Ficus carica)**- Figs have an interesting healing story found in the Bible from almost 3000 years ago. In the book of Isaiah chapter 38 verses 1,4, & 21, it tells the story of healing king Hezekiah. "In those days was Hezekiah **sick unto death**. And Isaiah the prophet the son of Amoz came unto him, and said unto him, Thus saith the LORD, Set thine house in order: for thou shalt die, and not live. Then came the word of the LORD to Isaiah, saying, For Isaiah had said, **Let them take a lump of figs**, and lay it for a plaster upon **the boil, and he shall recover**." Boils do not normally make people "sick unto death" so the word translated "boil" may have really meant "tumor", and coincidentally figs have now been scientifically studied to have anticancer properties. One study of fig extract showed that it "exhibited potent cytotoxicity in some human cancer cells with little effect in normal cells", in other words, selective cancer-cell killing.

AlGhalban FM, Khan AA, Khattak MNK. Comparative anticancer activities of *Ficus carica* and *Ficus salicifolia* latex in MDA-MB-231 cells. Saudi J Biol Sci. 2021 Jun;28(6):3225-3234. doi: 10.1016/j.sjbs.2021.02.061. Epub 2021 Feb 24. PMID: 34121859; PMCID: PMC8176001.

Soltana H, Pinon A, Limami Y, Zaid Y, Khalki L, Zaid N, Salah D, Sabitaliyevich UY, Simon A, Liagre B, Hammami M. Antitumoral activity of Ficus carica L. on colorectal cancer cell lines. Cell Mol Biol (Noisy-le-grand). 2019 Jul 31;65(6):6-11. PMID: 31472041.

Zhang Y, Wan Y, Huo B, Li B, Jin Y, Hu X. Extracts and components of *Ficus carica* leaves suppress survival, cell cycle, and migration of triple-negative breast cancer MDA-MB-231 cells. Onco Targets Ther. 2018 Jul 27;11:4377-4386. doi: 10.2147/OTT.S171601. PMID: 30100743; PMCID: PMC6067789.

**Flax Seeds (Linum usitatissimum)** - Flax seeds contain omega-3 fatty acids, lignans, and fiber, which can all help support healing the cancer process. Ground flax seed can help to lower breast and prostate cancer risk. Flax oil is one of the central components of the Budwig diet for cancer, which is a very healthy combination of flax oil and cottage cheese that contains most of the essential fats and proteins needed for human health.

Keykhasalar R, Tabrizi MH, Ardalan P, Khatamian N. The Apoptotic, Cytotoxic, and Antiangiogenic Impact of *Linum usitatissimum* Seed Essential Oil Nanoemulsions on the Human Ovarian Cancer Cell Line A2780. Nutr Cancer. 2021;73(11-12):2388-2396. doi: 10.1080/01635581.2020.1824001. Epub 2020 Sep 22. PMID: 32959696.

Jang WY, Kim MY, Cho JY. Antioxidant, Anti-Inflammatory, Anti-Menopausal, and Anti-Cancer Effects of Lignans and Their Metabolites. Int J Mol Sci. 2022 Dec 7;23(24):15482. doi: 10.3390/ijms232415482. PMID: 36555124; PMCID: PMC9778916.

Hazafa A, Iqbal MO, Javaid U, Tareen MBK, Amna D, Ramzan A, Piracha S, Naeem M. Inhibitory effect of polyphenols (phenolic acids, lignans, and stilbenes) on cancer by regulating signal transduction pathways: a review. Clin Transl Oncol. 2022 Mar;24(3):432-445. doi: 10.1007/s12094-021-02709-3. Epub 2021 Oct 5. PMID: 34609675.

**Garlic (Allium sativum)** - Has been used for cancers for at least 2,500 years. This well-known spice is a warming and drying food that has powerful antibacterial, antiviral, antifungal, and circulatory properties. It has been studied to slow cancer cell proliferation and induce apoptosis. It is extremely affordable and delicious in a vast number of recipes.

Rauf A, Abu-Izneid T, Thiruvengadam M, Imran M, Olatunde A, Shariati MA, Bawazeer S, Naz S, Shirooie S, Sanches-Silva A, Farooq U, Kazhybayeva G. Garlic (Allium sativum L.): Its Chemistry, Nutritional Composition, Toxicity, and Anticancer Properties. Curr Top Med Chem. 2022;22(11):957-972. doi: 10.2174/1568026621666211105094939. PMID: 34749610.

Mondal A, Banerjee S, Bose S, Mazumder S, Haber RA, Farzaei MH, Bishayee A. Garlic constituents for cancer prevention and therapy: From phytochemistry to novel formulations. Pharmacol Res. 2022 Jan;175:105837. doi: 10.1016/j.phrs.2021.105837. Epub 2021 Aug 24. PMID: 34450316.

Özkan İ, Koçak P, Yıldırım M, Ünsal N, Yılmaz H, Telci D, Şahin F. Garlic (Allium sativum)-derived SEVs inhibit cancer cell proliferation and induce caspase mediated apoptosis. Sci Rep. 2021 Jul 20;11(1):14773. doi: 10.1038/s41598-021-93876-4. PMID: 34285262; PMCID: PMC8292337.

**Ginger (Zingiber officinalis)**- This spicy Asian root has a bounty of medicinal properties. It acts as a double cancer therapy. It has direct anti-inflammatory and anti-cancer effects in triggering apoptosis and slowing cancer cell growth. And due to its famous properties for reducing nausea and vomiting it is used as a first aid to help reduce nausea from chemotherapy treatments. Ginger is available in many forms from natural ginger ale, to dried powder, to fresh grated root, to ginger chews, to fresh home-made juice in juicer recipes. It can add a delicious and healing spicy kick to many fresh fruit and vegetable juices.

Warin RF, Chen H, Soroka DN, Zhu Y, Sang S. Induction of lung cancer cell apoptosis through a p53 pathway by [6]-shogaol and its cysteine-conjugated metabolite M2. J Agric Food Chem. 2014 Feb 12;62(6):1352-62. doi: 10.1021/jf405573e. Epub 2014 Jan 30. PMID: 24446736; PMCID: PMC3983336.

Hafuth S, Randhawa S. Investigating the Anti-Cancer Properties of 6-Shogaol in Zingiber officinale. Crit Rev Oncog. 2022;27(3):15-22. doi: 10.1615/CritRevOncog.2022045100. PMID: 37183935.

Mega Tiber P, Kocyigit Sevinc S, Kilinc O, Orun O. Biological effects of whole Z.Officinale extract on chronic myeloid leukemia cell line K562. Gene. 2019 Apr 15;692:217-222. doi: 10.1016/j.gene.2019.01.015. Epub 2019 Jan 24. PMID: 30684525.

**Grapes (Vitis vinifera)-** The most medicinal parts of grapes are the skins and the seeds. So if you run grapes through a juicer and give away the juice, the leftover pulp is where all the anticancer molecules reside. These compounds include: anthocyanins, resveratrol, and other polyphenols. Resveratrol has a symphony of anticancer effects including all stages of initiation, promotion, and progression.

Grace Nirmala J, Evangeline Celsia S, Swaminathan A, Narendhirakannan RT, Chatterjee S. Cytotoxicity and apoptotic cell death induced by Vitis vinifera peel and seed extracts in A431 skin cancer cells. Cytotechnology. 2018 Apr;70(2):537-554. doi: 10.1007/s10616-017-0125-0. Epub 2017 Oct 5. PMID: 28983752; PMCID: PMC5851950.

Ferraz da Costa DC, Pereira Rangel L, Quarti J, Santos RA, Silva JL, Fialho E. Bioactive Compounds and Metabolites from Grapes and Red Wine in Breast Cancer Chemoprevention and Therapy. Molecules. 2020 Aug 1;25(15):3531. doi: 10.3390/molecules25153531. PMID: 32752302; PMCID: PMC7436232.

Kaur M, Agarwal C, Agarwal R. Anticancer and cancer chemopreventive potential of grape seed extract and other grape-based products. J Nutr. 2009 Sep;139(9):1806S-12S. doi: 10.3945/jn.109.106864. Epub 2009 Jul 29. PMID: 19640973; PMCID: PMC2728696.

**Green Tea (Camellia sinensis)-** Is one of the most famous and well-studied cancer fighters. Drink either organic green tea or green tea extract capsules daily. It is DNA protective, supports faster carcinogen removal from the body, and makes conventional chemo and radiation more effective. It has antiangiogenic, antioxidant, and antimitotic properties. The caffeine in tea even has some anticancer benefits. The most well-known molecule in green tea is Epigallocatechin Gallate (EGCG) which is denatured when green tea is converted into black tea.

Rafieian-Kopaei M, Movahedi M. Breast cancer chemopreventive and chemotherapeutic effects of Camellia Sinensis (green tea): an updated review. Electron Physician. 2017 Feb 25;9(2):3838-3844. doi: 10.19082/3838. PMID: 28465816; PMCID: PMC5410915.

Shirakami Y, Shimizu M. Possible Mechanisms of Green Tea and Its Constituents against Cancer. Molecules. 2018 Sep 7;23(9):2284. doi: 10.3390/molecules23092284. PMID: 30205425; PMCID: PMC6225266.

Filippini T, Malavolti M, Borrelli F, Izzo AA, Fairweather-Tait SJ, Horneber M, Vinceti M. Green tea (Camellia sinensis) for the prevention of cancer. Cochrane Database Syst Rev. 2020 Mar 2;3(3):CD005004. doi: 10.1002/14651858.CD005004.pub3. PMID: 32118296; PMCID: PMC7059963.

**Kiwi Berry (Actinidia arguta)-** Provides cancer-preventative and treatment molecules. These are smaller cousins of the supermarket kiwi that have smooth edible skins and they can even be found at Costco on occasion. They have been studied to trigger apoptosis in some cancer cells.

Nishimura M, Okimasu Y, Miyake N, Tada M, Hida R, Negishi T, Arimoto-Kobayashi S. Inhibitory effect of *Actinidia arguta* on mutagenesis, inflammation and two-stage mouse skin tumorigenesis. Genes Environ. 2016 Nov 1;38:25. doi: 10.1186/s41021-016-0053-9. PMID: 27822323; PMCID: PMC5088666.

Zhao X, Wen F, Wang W, Lu Z, Guo Q. Actinidia arguta (Hardy Kiwi) Root Extract Exerts Anti-cancer Effects via Mcl-1-Mediated Apoptosis in Cholangiocarcinoma. Nutr Cancer. 2019;71(2):246-256. doi: 10.1080/01635581.2018.1557218. Epub 2019 Jan 11. PMID: 30633583.

Lim S, Han SH, Kim J, Lee HJ, Lee JG, Lee EJ. Inhibition of hardy kiwifruit (Actinidia aruguta) ripening by 1-methylcyclopropene during cold storage and anticancer properties of the fruit extract. Food Chem. 2016 Jan 1;190:150-157. doi: 10.1016/j.foodchem.2015.05.085. Epub 2015 May 19. PMID: 26212954.

**Leeks (Allium porrum)**- This is a relative of garlic and onion that helps prevent prostate, colon, and ovarian cancers. Leeks and all of their cousins in the allium family (garlic, onion, leeks, chives, shallots) contain cancer-fighting sulfur molecules including: diallyl disulfide, dipropyl disulfide, and dimethyl disulfide, among many others.

Nicastro HL, Ross SA, Milner JA. Garlic and onions: their cancer prevention properties. Cancer Prev Res (Phila). 2015 Mar;8(3):181-9. doi: 10.1158/1940-6207.CAPR-14-0172. Epub 2015 Jan 13. PMID: 25586902; PMCID: PMC4366009.

Alam A, Al Arif Jahan A, Bari MS, Khandokar L, Mahmud MH, Junaid M, Chowdhury MS, Khan MF, Seidel V, Haque MA. Allium vegetables: Traditional uses, phytoconstituents, and beneficial effects in inflammation and cancer. Crit Rev Food Sci Nutr. 2023;63(23):6580-6614. doi: 10.1080/10408398.2022.2036094. Epub 2022 Feb 16. PMID: 35170391.

**Nutmeg (Myristica fragrans)**- This common spice contains the flavonoid myristicin that may be an effective cancer chemopreventive agent. Laboratory Studies have shown that it helps to inhibit an enzyme called lactate dehydrogenase (LDH) that cancer cells use to burn glucose for fuel. It can also trigger autophagy (self digesting) of cancer cells.

Kim EY, Choi HJ, Park MJ, Jung YS, Lee SO, Kim KJ, Choi JH, Chung TW, Ha KT. Myristica fragrans Suppresses Tumor Growth and Metabolism by Inhibiting Lactate Dehydrogenase A. Am J Chin Med. 2016;44(5):1063-79. doi: 10.1142/S0192415X16500592. Epub 2016 Jul 19. PMID: 27430914.

Li C, Zhang K, Pan G, Ji H, Li C, Wang X, Hu X, Liu R, Deng L, Wang Y, Yang L, Cui H. Dehydrodiisoeugenol inhibits colorectal cancer growth by endoplasmic reticulum stress-induced autophagic pathways. J Exp Clin Cancer Res. 2021 Apr 10;40(1):125. doi: 10.1186/s13046-021-01915-9. Erratum in: J Exp Clin Cancer Res. 2023 Jun 24;42(1):153. PMID: 33838688; PMCID: PMC8035743.

Chumkaew P, Srisawat T. New neolignans from the seeds of Myristica fragrans and their cytotoxic activities. J Nat Med. 2019 Jan;73(1):273-277. doi: 10.1007/s11418-018-1246-2. Epub 2018 Aug 30. PMID: 30168038.

**Oregano (Origanum vulgare)-** This kitchen spice contains carvacrol, thymol, and linalool, among other terpenes that have shown anti-cancer effects. Oregano is world famous for being a powerful antibacterial and antiviral plant. It has anti-inflammatory and immune-supporting effects as well.

Balusamy SR, Perumalsamy H, Huq MA, Balasubramanian B. Anti-proliferative activity of Origanum vulgare inhibited lipogenesis and induced mitochondrial mediated apoptosis in human stomach cancer cell lines. Biomed Pharmacother. 2018 Dec;108:1835-1844. doi: 10.1016/j.biopha.2018.10.028. Epub 2018 Oct 19. PMID: 30372889.

Emire Z, Yabalak E. Can Origanum be a hope for cancer treatment? A review on the potential of Origanum species in preventing and treating cancers. Int J Environ Health Res. 2023 Sep;33(9):894-910. doi: 10.1080/09603123.2022.2064437. Epub 2022 Apr 13. PMID: 35414316.

Begnini KR, Nedel F, Lund RG, Carvalho PH, Rodrigues MR, Beira FT, Del-Pino FA. Composition and antiproliferative effect of essential oil of Origanum vulgare against tumor cell lines. J Med Food. 2014 Oct;17(10):1129-33. doi: 10.1089/jmf.2013.0063. Epub 2014 Sep 17. PMID: 25230257.

**Parsley (Petroselinum crispum)-** Common parsley is a natural remedy for bad breath, digestion, and infections. It has powerful antioxidant, anti inflammatory, and anticancer effects. It contains flavonoids like myricetin and apigenin that have been studied for their DNA protective, cancer-growth slowing, and cancer-killing properties.

Tang EL, Rajarajeswaran J, Fung S, Kanthimathi MS. Petroselinum crispum has antioxidant properties, protects against DNA damage and inhibits proliferation and migration of cancer cells. J Sci Food Agric. 2015 Oct;95(13):2763-71. doi: 10.1002/jsfa.7078. Epub 2015 Feb 19. PMID: 25582089; PMCID: PMC5024025.

Aissani N, Albouchi F, Sebai H. Anticancer Effect in Human Glioblastoma and Antioxidant Activity of *Petroselinum crispum* L. Methanol Extract. Nutr Cancer. 2021;73(11-12):2605-2613. doi: 10.1080/01635581.2020.1842894. Epub 2020 Oct 29. PMID: 33121278.

Wu KH, Lee WJ, Cheng TC, Chang HW, Chen LC, Chen CC, Lien HM, Lin TN, Ho YS. Study of the antitumor mechanisms of apiole derivatives (AP-02) from Petroselinum crispum through induction of G0/G1 phase cell cycle arrest in human COLO 205 cancer cells. BMC Complement Altern Med. 2019 Jul 27;19(1):188. doi: 10.1186/s12906-019-2590-9. PMID: 31351461; PMCID: PMC6660667.

**Pomegranate (Punica granatum)-** This delicious fruit contains ellagic acid, phenols, and anthocyanins. It is most studied for prostate cancer. It suppresses inflammation, internal testosterone production. and down regulates T-receptors. It has been shown to reduce PSA doubling time by 50% and its molecules are known to concentrate in the male prostate gland.

Sharma P, McClees SF, Afaq F. Pomegranate for Prevention and Treatment of Cancer: An Update. Molecules. 2017 Jan 24;22(1):177. doi: 10.3390/molecules22010177. PMID: 28125044; PMCID: PMC5560105.

Moga MA, Dimienescu OG, Bălan A, Dima L, Toma SI, Bîgiu NF, Blidaru A. Pharmacological and Therapeutic Properties of *Punica granatum* Phytochemicals: Possible Roles in Breast Cancer. Molecules. 2021 Feb 17;26(4):1054. doi: 10.3390/molecules26041054. PMID: 33671442; PMCID: PMC7921999.

Sharma P, McClees SF, Afaq F. Pomegranate for Prevention and Treatment of Cancer: An Update. Molecules. 2017 Jan 24;22(1):177. doi: 10.3390/molecules22010177. PMID: 28125044; PMCID: PMC5560105.

**Raspberry (Rubus idaeus)**- These fruits are high in ellagic acid, ellagitannins, and anthocyanins that have anti-inflammatory and anticancer effects. They have been shown to inhibit the MMP enzymes that contribute to metastasis and invasion.

Huang YW, Chuang CY, Hsieh YS, Chen PN, Yang SF, Shih-Hsuan-Lin, Chen YY, Lin CW, Chang YC. Rubus idaeus extract suppresses migration and invasion of human oral cancer by inhibiting MMP-2 through modulation of the Erk1/2 signaling pathway. Environ Toxicol. 2017 Mar;32(3):1037-1046. doi: 10.1002/tox.22302. Epub 2016 Jun 20. PMID: 27322511.

Joubert KS, George BP, Razlog R, Abrahamse H. The In-Vitro Effect of Homeopathically Prepared Rubus idaeus and 680 nm Laser Irradiation on Cervical Cancer Cells. Homeopathy. 2023 Feb;112(1):50-56. doi: 10.1055/s-0042-1747683. Epub 2022 Jul 14. PMID: 35835442.

Hsieh YS, Chu SC, Hsu LS, Chen KS, Lai MT, Yeh CH, Chen PN. Rubus idaeus L. reverses epithelial-to-mesenchymal transition and suppresses cell invasion and protease activities by targeting ERK1/2 and FAK pathways in human lung cancer cells. Food Chem Toxicol. 2013 Dec;62:908-18. doi: 10.1016/j.fct.2013.10.021. Epub 2013 Oct 24. PMID: 24161487

**Rhubarb (Rheum species)**- This vegetable and its cousins contain anthraquinones, rhein, emodin, and aloe-emodin. It is used in Traditional Chinese Medicine for constipation, inflammation, and oxidation. It has anticancer and antimetastatic effects.

Huang Q, Lu G, Shen HM, Chung MC, Ong CN. Anti-cancer properties of anthraquinones from rhubarb. Med Res Rev. 2007 Sep;27(5):609-30. doi: 10.1002/med.20094. PMID: 17022020.

Chen YY, Hsieh MJ, Hsieh YS, Chang YC, Chen PN, Yang SF, Ho HY, Chou YE, Lin CW. Antimetastatic effects of Rheum palmatum L. extract on oral cancer cells. Environ Toxicol. 2017 Oct;32(10):2287-2294. doi: 10.1002/tox.22444. Epub 2017 Jul 5. PMID: 28678381.

Tan YR, Lu Y. Molecular mechanism of Rhubarb in the treatment of non-small cell lung cancer based on network pharmacology and molecular docking technology. Mol Divers. 2023 Jun;27(3):1437-1457. doi: 10.1007/s11030-022-10501-w. Epub 2022 Aug 6. PMID: 35933455.

**Rosemary (Rosmarinus officinalis)**- Contains many cancer-fighting molecules such as caffeic acid, rosmarinic acid, carnosic acid, ursolic acid, and carnosol. It also has powerful liver protective, memory protecting, and antioxidant effects.

Moore J, Yousef M, Tsiani E. Anticancer Effects of Rosemary (Rosmarinus officinalis L.) Extract and Rosemary Extract Polyphenols. Nutrients. 2016 Nov 17;8(11):731. doi: 10.3390/nu8110731. PMID: 27869665; PMCID: PMC5133115.

Allegra A, Tonacci A, Pioggia G, Musolino C, Gangemi S. Anticancer Activity of *Rosmarinus officinalis* L.: Mechanisms of Action and Therapeutic Potentials. Nutrients. 2020 Jun 10;12(6):1739. doi: 10.3390/nu12061739. PMID: 32532056; PMCID: PMC7352773.

Kakouri E, Nikola O, Kanakis C, Hatziagapiou K, Lambrou GI, Trigas P, Kanaka-Gantenbein C, Tarantilis PA. Cytotoxic Effect of *Rosmarinus officinalis* Extract on Glioblastoma and Rhabdomyosarcoma Cell Lines. Molecules. 2022 Sep 26;27(19):6348. doi: 10.3390/molecules27196348. PMID: 36234882; PMCID: PMC9573533.

**Saffron (Crocus sativus)**- The molecules safrole and crocin are thought to be the most important. It has been used for depression, and problems with the liver, kidneys, circulation, and menstruation. It works through various anticancer mechanisms including: regulation of tumor metabolism, cell-cycle progression, induction of apoptosis, and immune modulation.

Abdullaev FI. Cancer chemopreventive and tumoricidal properties of saffron (Crocus sativus L.). Exp Biol Med (Maywood). 2002 Jan;227(1):20-5. doi: 10.1177/153537020222700104. PMID: 11788779.

Khorasanchi Z, Shafiee M, Kermanshahi F, Khazaei M, Ryzhikov M, Parizadeh MR, Kermanshahi B, Ferns GA, Avan A, Hassanian SM. Crocus sativus a natural food coloring and flavoring has potent anti-tumor properties. Phytomedicine. 2018 Apr 1;43:21-27. doi: 10.1016/j.phymed.2018.03.041. Epub 2018 Mar 19. PMID: 29747750.

Bhandari PR. Crocus sativus L. (saffron) for cancer chemoprevention: A mini review. J Tradit Complement Med. 2015 Jan 28;5(2):81-7. doi: 10.1016/j.jtcme.2014.10.009. PMID: 26151016; PMCID: PMC4488115.

**Soy (Glycine max)**- Soybeans have been a massive topic of controversy in the cancer field for many years. Many oncologists have forbidden women with breast cancer to eat any soy products due to fears that they contain phytoestrogens that may be able to stimulate hormonal cancers. However, the research continues to show that soy and its isoflavones such as genistein and daidzein work more like tamoxifen which tends to block breast estrogen receptors. Soy extracts have proven anti-angiogenic, cell-growth reducing, and apoptosis inducing properties.

Bhat SS, Prasad SK, Shivamallu C, Prasad KS, Syed A, Reddy P, Cull CA, Amachawadi RG. Genistein: A Potent Anti-Breast Cancer Agent. Curr Issues Mol Biol. 2021 Oct 10;43(3):1502-1517. doi: 10.3390/cimb43030106. PMID: 34698063; PMCID: PMC8929066.

Douglas CC, Johnson SA, Arjmandi BH. Soy and its isoflavones: the truth behind the science in breast cancer. Anticancer Agents Med Chem. 2013 Oct;13(8):1178-87. doi: 10.2174/18715206113139990320. PMID: 23919747.

Varinska L, Gal P, Mojzisova G, Mirossay L, Mojzis J. Soy and breast cancer: focus on angiogenesis. Int J Mol Sci. 2015 May 22;16(5):11728-49. doi: 10.3390/ijms160511728. PMID: 26006245; PMCID: PMC4463727.

**Turmeric (Curcuma longa)**- This is one of the most studied anticancer foods on earth. It inhibits: tumor growth, antiapoptotic signals, and angiogenesis. It is a more powerful antioxidant than vitamin C. It inhibits the COX, LOX, and NFKB inflammation pathways. It has been used in India & China for thousands of years. It synergizes well with the pineapple enzyme bromelain for fibrinolytic therapy (breaking down the fibrin protein found in clots and scar tissue). Turmeric root powder is made more bioavailable when combined with fat and black pepper as it is in classic curry dishes.

Unlu A, Nayir E, Dogukan Kalenderoglu M, Kirca O, Ozdogan M. Curcumin (Turmeric) and cancer. J BUON. 2016 Sept-Oct;21(5):1050-1060. PMID: 27837604.

Nair A, Amalraj A, Jacob J, Kunnumakkara AB, Gopi S. Non-Curcuminoids from Turmeric and Their Potential in Cancer Therapy and Anticancer Drug Delivery Formulations. Biomolecules. 2019 Jan 2;9(1):13. doi: 10.3390/biom9010013. PMID: 30609771; PMCID: PMC6358877.

Fabianowska-Majewska K, Kaufman-Szymczyk A, Szymanska-Kolba A, Jakubik J, Majewski G, Lubecka K. Curcumin from Turmeric Rhizome: A Potential Modulator of DNA Methylation Machinery in Breast Cancer Inhibition. Nutrients. 2021 Jan 23;13(2):332. doi: 10.3390/nu13020332. PMID: 33498667; PMCID: PMC7910847.

## Foods With the Power To Kill Cancer Stem Cells

From the incredible natural health researcher and author, Sayer Ji, here are 25 of the top healing molecules found in foods and herbs that have been shown to kill cancer stem cells (these are the cells that float to other parts of the body and spread cancer elsewhere, and the ones that survive after chemo and radiation have blasted away the weaker 95% of the cancer cells.)

1. Epigallocatechin-3-gallate (EGCG) - **Green Tea**
2. 6-Gingerol - **Ginger**
3. β-Carotene - **Carrots, Sweet Potatoes, Leafy Greens**
4. Baicalein - **Chinese Skullcap**
5. Curcumin - **Turmeric**
6. Cyclopamine - Corn Lilly (we do not suggest consuming this plant; this simply illustrates natural components exist that kill cancer stem cells)
7. Delphinidin - **Blueberry, raspberry**
8. Genistein - **Soy, red clover**
9. Gossypol - Cottonseed (we do not suggest consuming this plant; this simply illustrates natural components exist that kill cancer stem cells)
10. Guggulsterone - **Myrrh & Guggul Herbs**
11. Isothiocyanates - **Cruciferous vegetables (Broccoli, Cauliflower, Cabbage, Mustard Greens, Brussels Sprouts, etc)**
12. Linalool - **Mint Family Herbs**
13. Lycopene - **Grapefruit, Tomato, Watermelon**
14. Parthenolide - **Feverfew**
15. Perylill alcohol - **Mint, Cherry, Lavender**
16. Piperine - **Black pepper**
17. Platycodon saponin - **Platycodon grandiflorum (a Chinese Herb)**
18. Psoralidin - **Psoralea corylilyfolia (Herb from China & India)**
19. Quercetin - **Capers, Onions, Apples, Berries**

20. Resveratrol - **Grapes, Plums, Berries**

21. Salinomycin - **Streptomyces albus (A Soil Bacteria)**

22. Silibinin - **Milk Thistle**

23. Ursolic acid - **Thyme, Basil, Oregano**

24. Vitamin D3 - **Sunshine, Fish, Egg yolk, Beef, Cod Liver Oil**

25. Withaferin A - **Withania somnifera (Ashwagandha)**

## Chapter 7 Action Steps

If you need more support for food choices, work with a Naturopathic Doctor, Certified Nutritionist, or Nutritional Health Coach near you.

- Write in your journal some of the new foods mentioned in this chapter that you would like to try soon.

- Go to RediscoverHealthNaturalMedicine.com to download your FREE copy of *Eating For Beating Cancer: Foods, Strategies, & Recipes To Increase Your Probability For Long-Term Health.*

## Resources

### Books:

**Keto for Cancer: Ketogenic Metabolic Therapy as a Targeted Nutritional Strategy** -Miriam Kalamian & Thomas Seyfried

**Beating Cancer with Nutrition** -Patrick Quillin

**The Longevity Diet** -Valter Longo

**Cancer as a metabolic disease: On the origin, management and prevention of cancer** -Thomas N. Seyfried

**Tripping over the Truth: How the Metabolic Theory of Cancer Is Overturning One of Medicine's Most Entrenched Paradigms** -Travis Christofferson

Eat to Beat Disease: The New Science of How Your Body Can Heal Itself
-William Li

## Websites:

https://greenmedinfo.com/blog/25-cancer-stem-cell-killing-foods-smarter-chemo-radiation2

## Videos:

**Angiogenesis and Foods-** http://youtube.com/watch?v=OjkzfeJz66o

# Chapter 8

## Molecular Pathway: Part 2- Herbal Medicine

"Herbal medicine assists healing through the sacred human-to-plant relationship."

-Donnie Yance -Best-Selling Author & Cancer Clinician

Here are some of the top 50 or so herbs that have scientific studies showing their anticancer properties. For convenience, they are listed in alphabetical order.

There wasn't enough room in this book to cover all of the herbs that my team and I researched, so if you would like to learn about even more of the anticancer herbs go to the bonus section of my website, **www.rediscoverhealthnaturalmedicine.com** for the rest of the list.

-A-

**American Ginseng (Panax quinquefolium)** - Has been studied to reverse cancer cells back to normal cells. It supports fatigue, mood, and memory. Studies suggest that compounds in American ginseng possess anti-tumor effects influencing cancer-cell growth and progression. Additionally, it's been investigated for its ability to boost the immune system, potentially aiding in cancer prevention and management.

Szczuka D, Nowak A, Zakłos-Szyda M, Kochan E, Szymańska G, Motyl I, Blasiak J. American Ginseng (*Panax quinquefolium* L.) as a Source of Bioactive Phytochemicals with Pro-Health Properties. Nutrients. 2019 May 9;11(5):1041. doi: 10.3390/nu11051041. PMID: 31075951; PMCID: PMC6567205.

Akhter KF, Mumin MA, Lui EMK, Charpentier PA. Transdermal nanotherapeutics: Panax quinquefolium polysaccharide nanoparticles attenuate UVB-induced skin cancer. Int J Biol Macromol. 2021 Jun 30;181:221-231. doi: 10.1016/j.ijbiomac.2021.03.122. Epub 2021 Mar 24. PMID: 33774070.

Kochan E, Nowak A, Zakłos-Szyda M, Szczuka D, Szymańska G, Motyl I. *Panax quinquefolium* L. Ginsenosides from Hairy Root Cultures and Their Clones Exert Cytotoxic, Genotoxic and Pro-Apoptotic Activity towards Human Colon Adenocarcinoma Cell Line Caco-2. Molecules. 2020 May 11;25(9):2262. doi: 10.3390/molecules25092262. PMID: 32403328; PMCID: PMC7249024.

**Andrographis (Andrographis paniculata)-** Research on Andrographis paniculata, commonly known as "King of Bitters," has unveiled potential anti-cancer properties attributed to its bioactive compounds. Studies indicate that this herb exhibits diverse effects, including anti-inflammatory, antioxidant, and immune-modulatory actions, which can impede cancer cell growth and metastasis. Additionally, Andrographis has been investigated for its ability to induce apoptosis (programmed cell death) in cancer cells, showing promise in inhibiting tumor progression in various cancer types. Some research suggests that its active components could potentially interfere with cancer cell signaling pathways and inhibit angiogenesis, the process of new blood vessel formation crucial for tumor growth. It is antiviral, inhibits cell proliferation, induces apoptosis, and causes G2/M cell phase arrest. It has kidney, nervous system, and liver-protective properties.

Dai Y, Chen SR, Chai L, Zhao J, Wang Y, Wang Y. Overview of pharmacological activities of *Andrographis paniculata* and its major compound andrographolide. Crit Rev Food Sci Nutr. 2019;59(sup1):S17-S29. doi: 10.1080/10408398.2018.1501657. Epub 2018 Sep 10. PMID: 30040451.

Cheung MK, Yue GG, Gomes AJ, Wong EC, Lee JK, Kwok FH, Chiu PW, Lau CB. Network pharmacology reveals potential functional components and underlying molecular mechanisms of Andrographis paniculata in esophageal cancer treatment. Phytother Res. 2022 Apr;36(4):1748-1760. doi: 10.1002/ptr.7411. Epub 2022 Feb 17. PMID: 35174914.

Wang XR, Jiang ZB, Xu C, Meng WY, Liu P, Zhang YZ, Xie C, Xu JY, Xie YJ, Liang TL, Yan HX, Fan XX, Yao XJ, Wu QB, Leung EL. Andrographolide suppresses non-small-cell lung cancer progression through induction of autophagy and antitumor immune response. Pharmacol Res. 2022 May;179:106198. doi: 10.1016/j.phrs.2022.106198. Epub 2022 Mar 31. PMID: 35367343.

**Angelica (Angelica archangelica)-** Research has highlighted anti-cancer properties attributed to its many bioactive compounds. Studies indicate that extracts from this plant exhibit various physiological effects, including antioxidant, anti-inflammatory, and anti-proliferative activities that impede cancer cell growth. Angelica archangelica has been investigated for its ability to induce apoptosis in certain cancer cells, showing potential in hindering tumor progression. Additionally, its active components have been studied for their potential to modulate immune responses, suggesting a role in enhancing the body's defense against cancerous cells.

It has been studied to support triple-negative breast, cervical, and laryngeal cancers.

Oliveira CR, Spindola DG, Garcia DM, Erustes A, Bechara A, Palmeira-Dos-Santos C, Smaili SS, Pereira GJS, Hinsberger A, Viriato EP, Cristina Marcucci M, Sawaya ACHF, Tomaz SL, Rodrigues EG, Bincoletto C. Medicinal properties of Angelica archangelica root extract: Cytotoxicity in breast cancer cells and its protective effects against in vivo tumor development. J Integr Med. 2019 Mar;17(2):132-140. doi: 10.1016/j.joim.2019.02.001. Epub 2019 Feb 8. PMID: 30799248.

Grabarska A, Skalicka-Woźniak K, Kiełbus M, Dmoszyńska-Graniczka M, Miziak P, Szumiło J, Nowosadzka E, Kowalczuk K, Khalifa S, Smok-Kalwat J, Klatka J, Kupisz K, Polberg K, Rivero-Müller A, Stepulak A. Imperatorin as a Promising Chemotherapeutic Agent Against Human Larynx Cancer and Rhabdomyosarcoma Cells. Molecules. 2020 Apr 28;25(9):2046. doi: 10.3390/molecules25092046. PMID: 32353989; PMCID: PMC7248852.

Sigurdsson S, Ogmundsdottir HM, Hallgrimsson J, Gudbjarnason S. Antitumour activity of Angelica archangelica leaf extract. In Vivo. 2005 Jan-Feb;19(1):191-4. PMID: 15796173.

**Ashwagandha (Withania somnifera)**- Has direct anti-cancer and immune-stimulating properties. It supports the body with the side effects of chemotherapy and radiation. It can increase the sensitivity of cancer cells to radiation therapy. Ashwagandha builds blood, and is known to increase white-blood-cell counts depleted from conventional treatments. This herb exhibits diverse effects, including antioxidant, anti-inflammatory, and immune-modulatory actions that can inhibit cancer cell proliferation and metastasis. It has been investigated for its ability to induce apoptosis, interfere with cancer-cell signaling pathways, and inhibit angiogenesis. It is unique for its ability to reduce stress and increase energy during the day while at the same time helping to support healthy sleep at night.

Paul S, Chakraborty S, Anand U, Dey S, Nandy S, Ghorai M, Saha SC, Patil MT, Kandimalla R, Proćków J, Dey A. Withania somnifera (L.) Dunal (Ashwagandha): A comprehensive review on ethnopharmacology, pharmacotherapeutics, biomedicinal and toxicological aspects. Biomed Pharmacother. 2021 Nov;143:112175. doi: 10.1016/j.biopha.2021.112175. Epub 2021 Sep 27. PMID: 34649336.

Mandlik Ingawale DS, Namdeo AG. Pharmacological evaluation of Ashwagandha highlighting its healthcare claims, safety, and toxicity aspects. J Diet Suppl. 2021;18(2):183-226. doi: 10.1080/19390211.2020.1741484. Epub 2020 Apr 3. PMID: 32242751.

Kashyap VK, Peasah-Darkwah G, Dhasmana A, Jaggi M, Yallapu MM, Chauhan SC. *Withania somnifera*: Progress towards a Pharmaceutical Agent for Immunomodulation and Cancer Therapeutics. Pharmaceutics. 2022 Mar 10;14(3):611. doi: 10.3390/pharmaceutics14030611. PMID: 35335986; PMCID: PMC8954542.

**Asparagus Root (Asparagus officinalis)**- This is the root of the common vegetable. Asparagus root contains phytochemicals such as saponins and flavonoids, exhibiting antioxidant and anti-inflammatory effects that can impede cancer cell proliferation. Additionally, asparagus extracts have been investigated for their ability to induce apoptosis and inhibit angiogenesis. It exhibits some anti-metastatic effects in various cancers.

Xu G, Kong W, Fang Z, Fan Y, Yin Y, Sullivan SA, Tran AQ, Clark LH, Sun W, Hao T, Zhao L, Zhou C, Bae-Jump VL. Asparagus officinalis Exhibits Anti-Tumorigenic and Anti-Metastatic Effects in Ovarian Cancer. Front Oncol. 2021 Jul 14;11:688461. doi: 10.3389/fonc.2021.688461. PMID: 34336674; PMCID: PMC8317209.

Zhang X, Wang J, Fan Y, Zhao Z, Paraghamian SE, Hawkins GM, Buckingham L, O'Donnell J, Hao T, Suo H, Yin Y, Sun W, Kong W, Sun D, Zhao L, Zhou C, Bae-Jump VL. Asparagus officinalis combined with paclitaxel exhibited synergistic anti-tumor activity in paclitaxel-sensitive and -resistant ovarian cancer cells. J Cancer Res Clin Oncol. 2022 Aug 25. doi: 10.1007/s00432-022-04276-8. Epub ahead of print. PMID: 36006482.

Romani A, Casciano F, Stevanin C, Maietti A, Tedeschi P, Secchiero P, Marchetti N, Voltan R. Anticancer Activity of Aqueous Extracts from *Asparagus officinalis* L. Byproduct on Breast Cancer Cells. Molecules. 2021 Oct 21;26(21):6369. doi: 10.3390/molecules26216369. PMID: 34770777; PMCID: PMC8588164.

**Astragalus (Astragalus membranaceus)**- This root has been used in China for thousands of years as a powerful immune enhancer. It can increase interferon, natural killer cells, and T cells, it's liver protective, inhibits platelet aggregation, and can increase strength and vitality. Astragalus contains saponins, flavonoids, and polysaccharides, exhibiting immunomodulatory, antioxidant, and anti-inflammatory effects that may hinder cancer cell proliferation and metastasis. Additionally, astragalus extracts have been investigated for their ability to induce apoptosis, interfere with cancer cell signaling pathways, and reduce the angiogenesis process.

Auyeung KK, Han QB, Ko JK. Astragalus membranaceus: A Review of its Protection Against Inflammation and Gastrointestinal Cancers. Am J Chin Med. 2016;44(1):1-22. doi: 10.1142/S0192415X16500014. PMID: 26916911.

Bian Y, Wang G, Zhou J, Yin G, Liu T, Liang L, Yang X, Zhang W, Ni K, Tang D, Yu Y. Astragalus membranaceus (Huangqi) and Rhizoma curcumae (Ezhu) decoction suppresses colorectal cancer via downregulation of Wnt5/β-Catenin signal. Chin Med. 2022 Jan 6;17(1):11. doi: 10.1186/s13020-021-00564-6. PMID: 34991661; PMCID: PMC8740427.

Zhang J, Wu C, Gao L, Du G, Qin X. Astragaloside IV derived from Astragalus membranaceus: A research review on the pharmacological effects. Adv Pharmacol. 2020;87:89-112. doi: 10.1016/bs.apha.2019.08.002. Epub 2019 Dec 18. PMID: 32089240.

-B-

**Baikal skullcap (Scutellaria baicalensis)**- This herb has antiviral effects by inhibiting the reverse transcriptase enzyme. It has been shown to promote cancer cell death in multiple cell types, and it is also anti inflammatory and immune supporting. Baikal contains flavonoids, particularly baicalein and baicalin, demonstrating antioxidant, anti-inflammatory, and anti-proliferative effects that slow cancer cell growth and metastasis.It has been studied for its ability to induce apoptosis, and slowing angiogenesis.

Alsharairi NA. *Scutellaria baicalensis* and Their Natural Flavone Compounds as Potential Medicinal Drugs for the Treatment of Nicotine-Induced Non-Small-Cell Lung Cancer and Asthma. Int J Environ Res Public Health. 2021 May 14;18(10):5243. doi: 10.3390/ijerph18105243. PMID: 34069141; PMCID: PMC8155851.

Cheng CS, Chen J, Tan HY, Wang N, Chen Z, Feng Y. Scutellaria baicalensis and Cancer Treatment: Recent Progress and Perspectives in Biomedical and Clinical Studies. Am J Chin Med. 2018;46(1):25-54. doi: 10.1142/S0192415X18500027. Epub 2018 Jan 9. PMID: 29316796.

Xiang L, Gao Y, Chen S, Sun J, Wu J, Meng X. Therapeutic potential of Scutellaria baicalensis Georgi in lung cancer therapy. Phytomedicine. 2022 Jan;95:153727. doi: 10.1016/j.phymed.2021.153727. Epub 2021 Sep 4. PMID: 34535372.

**Bilberry (Vaccinium myrtillus)**- These relatives of the blueberry and cranberry contain anthocyanosides, catechin, epicatechin, and oligomeric procyanidins. Many of these molecules have been studied for their anti-cancer effects including: blocking angiogenesis, growth inhibition, antioxidant, and anti-inflammatory actions.

Del Bubba M, Di Serio C, Renai L, Scordo CVA, Checchini L, Ungar A, Tarantini F, Bartoletti R. Vaccinium myrtillus L. extract and its native polyphenol-recombined mixture have anti-proliferative and pro-apoptotic effects on human prostate cancer cell lines. Phytother Res. 2021 Feb;35(2):1089-1098. doi: 10.1002/ptr.6879. Epub 2020 Sep 14. PMID: 32929801.

Katsube N, Iwashita K, Tsushida T, Yamaki K, Kobori M. Induction of apoptosis in cancer cells by Bilberry (Vaccinium myrtillus) and the anthocyanins. J Agric Food Chem. 2003 Jan 1;51(1):68-75. doi: 10.1021/jf025781x. PMID: 12502387.

**Birch (Betula alba)**- Birch trees contain betulinic acid which has been studied for its anticancer properties. People have used birch bark tea and birch sap for hundreds of years to detox and purify the body. Betulinic acid

has been studied to induce apoptosis, slow migration, and inhibit cancer cell duplication. More betulinic acid is found in the bark than in any other part such as the roots or leaves, so birch bark tea is a great form to take it in.

Rzeski W, Stepulak A, Szymański M, Sifringer M, Kaczor J, Wejksza K, Zdzisińska B, Kandefer-Szerszeń M. Betulinic acid decreases expression of bcl-2 and cyclin D1, inhibits proliferation, migration and induces apoptosis in cancer cells. Naunyn Schmiedebergs Arch Pharmacol. 2006 Oct;374(1):11-20. doi: 10.1007/s00210-006-0090-1. Epub 2006 Sep 9. PMID: 16964520.

Szoka L, Nazaruk J, Stocki M, Isidorov V. Santin and cirsimaritin from Betula pubescens and Betula pendula buds induce apoptosis in human digestive system cancer cells. J Cell Mol Med. 2021 Dec;25(24):11085-11096. doi: 10.1111/jcmm.17031. Epub 2021 Nov 9. PMID: 34755444; PMCID: PMC8650031.

Isidorov V, Szoka Ł, Nazaruk J. Cytotoxicity of white birch bud extracts: Perspectives for therapy of tumours. PLoS One. 2018 Aug 14;13(8):e0201949. doi: 10.1371/journal.pone.0201949. PMID: 30106978; PMCID: PMC6091957.

**Black Cumin (Nigella sativa)** - One of black cumin's most studied molecules is Thymoquinone, it shows anti-cancer activity by interfering with cancer cell DNA, blocking cancer-signaling molecules, and modulating the immune system, it has shown powerful anti-cancer effects in many types of cancer including: bladder, bone, breast, colon, gastric, lung, prostate, and ovarian.

Korak T, Ergül E, Sazci A. Nigella sativa and Cancer: A Review Focusing on Breast Cancer, Inhibition of Metastasis and Enhancement of Natural Killer Cell Cytotoxicity. Curr Pharm Biotechnol. 2020;21(12):1176-1185. doi: 10.2174/1389201021666200430120453. PMID: 32351178.

Ansary J, Giampieri F, Forbes-Hernandez TY, Regolo L, Quinzi D, Gracia Villar S, Garcia Villena E, Tutusaus Pifarre K, Alvarez-Suarez JM, Battino M, Cianciosi D. Nutritional Value and Preventive Role of *Nigella sativa* L. and Its Main Component Thymoquinone in Cancer: An Evidenced-Based Review of Preclinical and Clinical Studies. Molecules. 2021 Apr 7;26(8):2108. doi: 10.3390/molecules26082108. PMID: 33916916; PMCID: PMC8067617.

Almatroodi SA, Almatroudi A, Alsahli MA, Khan AA, Rahmani AH. Thymoquinone, an Active Compound of Nigella sativa: Role in Prevention and Treatment of Cancer. Curr Pharm Biotechnol. 2020;21(11):1028-1041. doi: 10.2174/1389201021666200416092743. PMID: 32297580.

**Black Raspberry (Rubus occidentalis)**- This deeply-pigmented berry contains ellagic acid, anthocyanins, and other flavonoids with anti-cancer and antioxidant properties. It has been shown to inhibit angiogenesis and slow cancer cell proliferation for many types of cancer.

Kula M, Krauze-Baranowska M. Rubus occidentalis: The black raspberry--its potential in the prevention of cancer. Nutr Cancer. 2016;68(1):18-28. doi: 10.1080/01635581.2016.1115095. Epub 2015 Dec 23. PMID: 26699735.

Johnson JL, Bomser JA, Scheerens JC, Giusti MM. Effect of black raspberry ( Rubus occidentalis L.) extract variation conditioned by cultivar, production site, and fruit maturity stage on colon cancer cell proliferation. J Agric Food Chem. 2011 Mar 9;59(5):1638-45. doi: 10.1021/jf1023388. Epub 2011 Feb 1. PMID: 21284384.

Liu Z, Schwimer J, Liu D, Greenway FL, Anthony CT, Woltering EA. Black raspberry extract and fractions contain angiogenesis inhibitors. J Agric Food Chem. 2005 May 18;53(10):3909-15. doi: 10.1021/jf048585u. PMID: 15884816.

**Burdock (Arctium lappa)**- A staple in many of the traditional cancer formulas (Hoxey, Essiac, Dr Christopher, etc) It helps cleanse and detoxify all cells. It has some direct anti-cancer properties. It contains benzaldehyde that has known anticancer properties, and a substance called B-factor that protects cells from mutation. Burdock root also helps reduce cancer-induced cachexia (muscle wasting) by slowing this unhealthy weight loss.

Taleb Agha M, Baharetha HM, Al-Mansoub MA, Tabana YM, Kaz Abdul Aziz NH, Yam MF, Abdul Majid AMS. Proapoptotic and Antiangiogenic Activities of *Arctium Lappa* L. on Breast Cancer Cell Lines. Scientifica (Cairo). 2020 May 17;2020:7286053. doi: 10.1155/2020/7286053. PMID: 32509375; PMCID: PMC7254072.

Han YH, Mun JG, Jeon HD, Yoon DH, Choi BM, Kee JY, Hong SH. The Extract of *Arctium lappa* L. Fruit (Arctii Fructus) Improves Cancer-Induced Cachexia by Inhibiting Weight Loss of Skeletal Muscle and Adipose Tissue. Nutrients. 2020 Oct 19;12(10):3195. doi: 10.3390/nu12103195. PMID: 33086629; PMCID: PMC7603378.

-C-

**Cat's Claw (Uncaria tomentosa)**- Also known as Una de Gato, it enhances the immune system and white blood cells. It has powerful anti-inflammatory, antioxidant, and anti-tumor properties. It has been shown to enhance DNA repair and is known to help inhibit the lactate dehydrogenase enzyme that cancer cells use to create energy so it can assist in the starvation of cancer cells.

Kośmider A, Czepielewska E, Kuraś M, Gulewicz K, Pietrzak W, Nowak R, Nowicka G. Uncaria tomentosa Leaves Decoction Modulates Differently ROS Production in Cancer and Normal Cells, and Effects Cisplatin Cytotoxicity. Molecules. 2017 Apr 12;22(4):620. doi: 10.3390/molecules22040620. PMID: 28417940; PMCID: PMC6154711.

Zari A, Alfarteesh H, Buckner C, Lafrenie R. Treatment with *Uncaria tomentosa* Promotes Apoptosis in B16-BL6 Mouse Melanoma Cells and Inhibits the Growth of B16-BL6 Tumours. Molecules. 2021 Feb 18;26(4):1066. doi: 10.3390/molecules26041066. PMID: 33670520; PMCID: PMC7922471.

Núñez C, Lozada-Requena I, Ysmodes T, Zegarra D, Saldaña F, Aguilar J. Nmunomodulación de Uncaria tomentosa sobre células dendríticas, il-12 y perfil TH1/TH2/TH17 en cáncer de mama [Immunomodulation of Uncaria tomentosa over dendritic cells, il-12 and profile TH1/TH2/TH17 in breast cancer]. Rev Peru Med Exp Salud Publica. 2015 Oct;32(4):643-51. Spanish. PMID: 26732910.

**Cleavers (Galium aparine)**- This herb is a soothing, cooling, diuretic, and helps with lymphatic function and detoxification. It has demonstrated anti-tumor actions including the induction of apoptosis and necrosis (cell death) in breast cancer cells.

Atmaca H, Bozkurt E, Cittan M, Dilek Tepe H. Effects of Galium aparine extract on the cell viability, cell cycle and cell death in breast cancer cell lines. J Ethnopharmacol. 2016 Jun 20;186:305-310. doi: 10.1016/j.jep.2016.04.007. Epub 2016 Apr 13. PMID: 27085941.

Schmidt M, Polednik C, Roller J, Hagen R. Galium verum aqueous extract strongly inhibits the motility of head and neck cancer cell lines and protects mucosal keratinocytes against toxic DNA damage. Oncol Rep. 2014 Sep;32(3):1296-302. doi: 10.3892/or.2014.3316. Epub 2014 Jul 9. PMID: 25017936.

**Codonopsis (Codonopsis pilosula)**- This Chinese herb also known as Dang Shen, has the power to stimulate macrophages, neutrophils, and T-cells of the immune system. It can renew red-blood cells in anemic conditions caused by cancer treatments. It increases energy and stamina, and has been used as a substitute for the more expensive ginseng root for hundreds of years. Extracts have been shown to slow cancer cell proliferation and metastasis.

Chen M, Li Y, Liu Z, Qu Y, Zhang H, Li D, Zhou J, Xie S, Liu M. Exopolysaccharides from a Codonopsis pilosula endophyte activate macrophages and inhibit cancer cell proliferation and migration. Thorac Cancer. 2018 May;9(5):630-639. doi: 10.1111/1759-7714.12630. Epub 2018 Mar 25. PMID: 29577649; PMCID: PMC5928371.

Hu N, Gao Z, Cao P, Song H, Hu J, Qiu Z, Chang C, Zheng G, Shan X, Meng Y. Uniform and disperse selenium nanoparticles stabilized by inulin fructans from Codonopsis pilosula and their anti-hepatoma activities. Int J Biol Macromol. 2022 Apr 1;203:105-115. doi: 10.1016/j.ijbiomac.2022.01.140. Epub 2022 Jan 29. PMID: 35092739.

Liu Z, Sun Y, Zhen H, Nie C. Network Pharmacology Integrated with Transcriptomics Deciphered the Potential Mechanism of Codonopsis pilosula against Hepatocellular Carcinoma. Evid Based Complement Alternat Med. 2022 Mar 27;2022:1340194. doi: 10.1155/2022/1340194. PMID: 35388300; PMCID: PMC8977304.

-D-

**Dandelion (Taraxicum officinalis)**- This common weed is also a powerful medicine. The flowers are edible and nutritious and the greens can be used in salads. Dandelion root has been historically used for breast and other cancers. It is a traditional liver remedy and enhances bile flow. It is rich in many nutrients and can be used as food or medicine. Studies have shown its ability to reduce the growth of cancer cells and induce apoptosis.

Wang S, Hao HF, Jiao YN, Fu JL, Guo ZW, Guo Y, Yuan Y, Li PP, Han SY. Dandelion extract inhibits triple-negative breast cancer cell proliferation by interfering with glycerophospholipids and unsaturated fatty acids metabolism. Front Pharmacol. 2022 Sep 6;13:942996. doi: 10.3389/fphar.2022.942996. PMID: 36147318; PMCID: PMC9486077.

Zhu H, Zhao H, Zhang L, Xu J, Zhu C, Zhao H, Lv G. Dandelion root extract suppressed gastric cancer cells proliferation and migration through targeting lncRNA-CCAT1. Biomed Pharmacother. 2017 Sep;93:1010-1017. doi: 10.1016/j.biopha.2017.07.007. Epub 2017 Jul 14. PMID: 28724210.

Nguyen C, Mehaidli A, Baskaran K, Grewal S, Pupulin A, Ruvinov I, Scaria B, Parashar K, Vegh C, Pandey S. Dandelion Root and Lemongrass Extracts Induce Apoptosis, Enhance Chemotherapeutic Efficacy, and Reduce Tumour Xenograft Growth *In Vivo* in Prostate Cancer. Evid Based Complement Alternat Med. 2019 Jul 17;2019:2951428. doi: 10.1155/2019/2951428. PMID: 31391857; PMCID: PMC6662490.

**Dan Shen (Salvia miltiorrhiza)**- This Chinese herb has many anticancer functions including: inducing apoptosis, blocking estrogen for some hormone-dependent cancers, blocking the MMP enzymes that dissolve connective tissue to spread metastasis, and blocking cancer-cell adhesion.

Zhou J, Jiang YY, Chen H, Wu YC, Zhang L. Tanshinone I attenuates the malignant biological properties of ovarian cancer by inducing apoptosis and autophagy via the inactivation of PI3K/AKT/mTOR pathway. Cell Prolif. 2020 Feb;53(2):e12739. doi: 10.1111/cpr.12739. Epub 2019 Dec 9. PMID: 31820522; PMCID: PMC7046305.

Lu M, Lan X, Wu X, Fang X, Zhang Y, Luo H, Gao W, Wu D. *Salvia miltiorrhiza* in cancer: Potential role in regulating MicroRNAs and epigenetic enzymes. Front Pharmacol. 2022 Sep 12;13:1008222. doi: 10.3389/fphar.2022.1008222. PMID: 36172186; PMCID: PMC9512245.

Zhao H, Han B, Li X, Sun C, Zhai Y, Li M, Jiang M, Zhang W, Liang Y, Kai G. *Salvia miltiorrhiza* in Breast Cancer Treatment: A Review of Its Phytochemistry, Derivatives, Nanoparticles, and Potential Mechanisms. Front Pharmacol. 2022 May 5;13:872085. doi: 10.3389/fphar.2022.872085. PMID: 35600860; PMCID: PMC9117704

-E-

**Echinacea (Echinacea angustifolia)**- This plant is world famous for stimulating the immune system, improving lymphatic function, increasing NK cell activity, boosting interferon, and activating T-cells. It also blocks an enzyme called hyaluronidase that dissolves connective tissue so it may slow the spread of cancer through metastasis. It has been shown to slow cancer cell growth and induce apoptosis and magnify the anti-cancer effects of some chemotherapy drugs including Paclitaxel.

Aarland RC, Bañuelos-Hernández AE, Fragoso-Serrano M, Sierra-Palacios ED, Díaz de León-Sánchez F, Pérez-Flores LJ, Rivera-Cabrera F, Mendoza-Espinoza JA. Studies on phytochemical, antioxidant, anti-inflammatory, hypoglycaemic and antiproliferative activities of Echinacea purpurea and Echinacea angustifolia extracts. Pharm Biol. 2017 Dec;55(1):649-656. doi: 10.1080/13880209.2016.1265989. PMID: 27951745; PMCID: PMC6130640.

Espinosa-Paredes DA, Cornejo-Garrido J, Moreno-Eutimio MA, Martínez-Rodríguez OP, Jaramillo-Flores ME, Ordaz-Pichardo C. Echinacea Angustifolia DC Extract Induces Apoptosis and Cell Cycle Arrest and Synergizes with Paclitaxel in the MDA-MB-231 and MCF-7 Human Breast Cancer Cell Lines. Nutr Cancer. 2021;73(11-12):2287-2305. doi: 10.1080/01635581.2020.1817956. Epub 2020 Sep 22. PMID: 32959676.

**Eleuthero (Eleutherococcus senticosus)**- This plant is also known as 'Siberian Ginseng' but it is not related to the ginseng family at all, so I will refer to it as Eleuthero here. It is a great adaptogen that improves the body's response to physical work, stress, fatigue, and chronic disease. Eleuthero extracts have been shown to induce apoptosis in cancer cells. It is also a fantastic support for those undergoing chemotherapy or radiation treatments.

Cichello SA, Yao Q, Dowell A, Leury B, He XQ. Proliferative and Inhibitory Activity of Siberian ginseng (Eleutherococcus senticosus) Extract on Cancer Cell Lines; A-549, XWLC-05, HCT-116, CNE and Beas-2b. Asian Pac J Cancer Prev. 2015;16(11):4781-6. doi: 10.7314/apjcp.2015.16.11.4781. PMID: 26107240.

Kim CG, Castro-Aceituno V, Abbai R, Lee HA, Simu SY, Han Y, Hurh J, Kim YJ, Yang DC. Caspase-3/MAPK pathways as main regulators of the apoptotic effect of the phyto-mediated synthesized silver nanoparticle from dried stem of Eleutherococcus senticosus in human cancer cells. Biomed Pharmacother. 2018 Mar;99:128-133. doi: 10.1016/j.biopha.2018.01.050. Epub 2018 Jan 10. PMID: 29331758.

-F-

**Feverfew (Tanacetum parthenium)** - This herb is most commonly used as a migraine headache remedy. However one of its molecules, parthenolide, also exhibits multiple anticancer and anti-inflammatory effects.

Dong Y, Qian X, Li J. Sesquiterpene Lactones and Cancer: New Insight into Antitumor and Anti-inflammatory Effects of Parthenolide-Derived Dimethylaminomicheliolide and Micheliolide. Comput Math Methods Med. 2022 Jul 18;2022:3744837. doi: 10.1155/2022/3744837. PMID: 35898475; PMCID: PMC9313921.

Mathema VB, Koh YS, Thakuri BC, Sillanpää M. Parthenolide, a sesquiterpene lactone, expresses multiple anti-cancer and anti-inflammatory activities. Inflammation. 2012 Apr;35(2):560-5. doi: 10.1007/s10753-011-9346-0. PMID: 21603970.

Berdan CA, Ho R, Lehtola HS, To M, Hu X, Huffman TR, Petri Y, Altobelli CR, Demeulenaere SG, Olzmann JA, Maimone TJ, Nomura DK. Parthenolide Covalently Targets and Inhibits Focal Adhesion Kinase in Breast Cancer Cells. Cell Chem Biol. 2019 Jul 18;26(7):1027-1035.e22. doi: 10.1016/j.chembiol.2019.03.016. Epub 2019 May 9. PMID: 31080076; PMCID: PMC6756182.

**Figwort (Scrophularia species)**- This herb is commonly used for mild pain, detoxification, and increased circulation. It has a special affinity for breast tissue, so it has been used traditionally for breast cancer. Several Scrophularia species have been studied for their ability to induce apoptosis and amplify the anticancer effects of chemo drugs such as Doxorubicin.

Safavi R, Soltanzadeh H, Hojjati Bonab Z. Scrophularia amplexicaulis increases anti-cancer potential of doxorubicin in gastric cancer cells. Environ Toxicol. 2023 Nov;38(11):2741-2750. doi: 10.1002/tox.23909. Epub 2023 Jul 20. PMID: 37471627.

Azadmehr A, Hajiaghaee R, Baradaran B, Haghdoost-Yazdi H. Apoptosis Cell Death Effect of Scrophularia Variegata on Breast Cancer Cells via Mitochondrial Intrinsic Pathway. Adv Pharm Bull. 2015 Sep;5(3):443-6. doi: 10.15171/apb.2015.060. Epub 2015 Sep 19. PMID: 26504768; PMCID: PMC4616888.

Ardeshiry Lajimi A, Rezaie-Tavirani M, Mortazavi SA, Barzegar M, Moghadamnia SH, Rezaee MB. Study of Anti Cancer Property of Scrophularia striata Extract on the Human Astrocytoma Cell Line (1321). Iran J Pharm Res. 2010 Fall;9(4):403-10. PMID: 24381605; PMCID: PMC3870064.

**Frankincense (Boswellia serrata, carterii, ovalifoliolata, & thurifera)-**
This ancient herb can increase cancer-cell apoptosis. It has been shown to increase chemo sensitivity in cancer cells, but not healthy cells. It decreases inflammation by lowering NFKB, 5-LOX, and other enzymes. Petroleum ether and methanol are the strongest types of extracts. It has been studied to support brain cancer and brain swelling as it can cross the blood-brain barrier to access the brain cells more directly.

Efferth T, Oesch F. Anti-inflammatory and anti-cancer activities of frankincense: Targets, treatments and toxicities. Semin Cancer Biol. 2022 May;80:39-57. doi: 10.1016/j.semcancer.2020.01.015. Epub 2020 Feb 4. PMID: 32027979.

Thummuri D, Jeengar MK, Shrivastava S, Areti A, Yerra VG, Yamjala S, Komirishetty P, Naidu VG, Kumar A, Sistla R. Boswellia ovalifoliolata abrogates ROS mediated NF-κB activation, causes apoptosis and chemosensitization in Triple Negative Breast Cancer cells. Environ Toxicol Pharmacol. 2014 Jul;38(1):58-70. doi: 10.1016/j.etap.2014.05.002. Epub 2014 May 14. PMID: 24908637.

Yazdanpanahi N, Behbahani M, Yektaeian A. Effect of boswellia thurifera gum methanol extract on cytotoxicity and p53 gene expression in human breast cancer cell line. Iran J Pharm Res. 2014 Spring;13(2):719-24. PMID: 25237368; PMCID: PMC4157048.

-G-

**Ginkgo (Ginkgo biloba)-** While Ginkgo is most famous for its memory-enhancing effects through increasing brain circulation, it can enhance the cancer-killing effects of chemo and radiation, as well as improve the immune system, make the blood more fluid, and decrease inflammation.

Lou JS, Zhao LP, Huang ZH, Chen XY, Xu JT, Tai WC, Tsim KWK, Chen YT, Xie T. Ginkgetin derived from Ginkgo biloba leaves enhances the therapeutic effect of cisplatin via ferroptosis-mediated disruption of the Nrf2/HO-1 axis in EGFR wild-type non-small-cell lung cancer. Phytomedicine. 2021 Jan;80:153370. doi: 10.1016/j.phymed.2020.153370. Epub 2020 Oct 9. PMID: 33113504.

Feodorova Y, Tomova T, Minchev D, Turiyski V, Draganov M, Argirova M. Cytotoxic effect of *Ginkgo biloba* kernel extract on HCT116 and A2058 cancer cell lines. Heliyon. 2020 Sep 19;6(9):e04941. doi: 10.1016/j.heliyon.2020.e04941. PMID: 33005784; PMCID: PMC7509470.

Fu Z, Lin L, Liu S, Qin M, He S, Zhu L, Huang J. Ginkgo Biloba Extract Inhibits Metastasis and ERK/Nuclear Factor kappa B (NF-κB) Signaling Pathway in Gastric Cancer. Med Sci Monit. 2019 Sep 11;25:6836-6845. doi: 10.12659/MSM.915146. PMID: 31509521; PMCID: PMC6753842.

**Ginseng (Panax ginseng)-** This herb enhances healing post surgery while also blocking metastasis. There are over 40 known ginsenosides that have direct anti-cancer, vitality improving, stress reducing, and anti-inflammatory actions. It helps optimize and heal from radiation therapy.

Zhou X, Liu H, Zhang M, Li C, Li G. Spectrum-effect relationship between UPLC fingerprints and anti-lung cancer effect of Panax ginseng. Phytochem Anal. 2021 May;32(3):339-346. doi: 10.1002/pca.2980. Epub 2020 Aug 18. PMID: 32808367; PMCID: PMC8048684.

Helms S. Cancer prevention and therapeutics: Panax ginseng. Altern Med Rev. 2004 Sep;9(3):259-74. PMID: 15387718.

Shin HR, Kim JY, Yun TK, Morgan G, Vainio H. The cancer-preventive potential of Panax ginseng: a review of human and experimental evidence. Cancer Causes Control. 2000 Jul;11(6):565-76. doi: 10.1023/a:1008980200583. PMID: 10880039.

**Goji Berries (Lycium barbarum)**- Goji, also known as olfberries, are a fruit that has been used in traditional Chinese medicine for thousands of years. Some of the benefits of goji berries include: they are rich in nutrients & antioxidants, support healthy blood glucose levels, antiinflammatory actions, support the immune system, and may protect against UV radiation.
Goji's anticancer properties include: inducing ferroptosis (iron-dependent cancer cell death), inhibition of migration, adhesion, and triggering apoptosis.

DU X, Zhang J, Liu L, Xu B, Han H, Dai W, Pei X, Fu X, Hou S. A novel anticancer property of *Lycium barbarum* polysaccharide in triggering ferroptosis of breast cancer cells. J Zhejiang Univ Sci B. 2022 Apr 15;23(4):286-299. English. doi: 10.1631/jzus.B2100748. PMID: 35403384; PMCID: PMC9002246.

Sanghavi A, Srivatsa A, Adiga D, Chopra A, Lobo R, Kabekkodu SP, Gadag S, Nayak U, Sivaraman K, Shah A. Goji berry (Lycium barbarum) inhibits the proliferation, adhesion, and migration of oral cancer cells by inhibiting the ERK, AKT, and CyclinD cell signaling pathways: an in-vitro study. F1000Res. 2022 Dec 22;11:1563. doi: 10.12688/f1000research.129250.3. PMID: 36761830; PMCID: PMC9887205.

Gong G, Liu Q, Deng Y, Dang T, Dai W, Liu T, Liu Y, Sun J, Wang L, Liu Y, Sun T, Song S, Wang Z, Huang L. Arabinogalactan derived from Lycium barbarum fruit inhibits cancer cell growth via cell cycle arrest and apoptosis. Int J Biol Macromol. 2020 Apr 15;149:639-650. doi: 10.1016/j.ijbiomac.2020.01.251. Epub 2020 Jan 25. PMID: 31991207.

**Goldenseal (Hydrastis canadensis)**- This herb has a high berberine content and has been used for colds and flus for hundreds of years. Newer studies show berberine as a molecule with glucose lowering, anti-inflammatory, and anticancer properties. In combination with cisplatin, berberine has been shown to synergize to create an even greater level of apoptosis.

Karmakar SR, Biswas SJ, Khuda-Bukhsh AR. Anti-carcinogenic potentials of a plant extract (Hydrastis canadensis): I. Evidence from in vivo studies in mice (Mus musculus). Asian Pac J Cancer Prev. 2010;11(2):545-51. PMID: 20843149.

Zhao Y, Jing Z, Li Y, Mao W. Berberine in combination with cisplatin suppresses breast cancer cell growth through induction of DNA breaks and caspase-3-dependent apoptosis. Oncol Rep. 2016 Jul;36(1):567-72. doi: 10.3892/or.2016.4785. Epub 2016 May 5. PMID: 27177238.

Guo B, Li X, Song S, Chen M, Cheng M, Zhao D, Li F. (-)-β-hydrastine suppresses the proliferation and invasion of human lung adenocarcinoma cells by inhibiting PAK4 kinase activity. Oncol Rep. 2016 Apr;35(4):2246-56. doi: 10.3892/or.2016.4594. Epub 2016 Jan 25. PMID: 26821251.

**Gotu Kola (Centella asiatica)**- Gotu Kola blocks protease enzymes that help cancer spread through connective tissues. It also supports wound healing, reduction of scar tissue, and promotes mental focus and memory. Centella provides some protection against radiation, and reduces inflammatory cytokines that can contribute to cancer cachexia.

Han AR, Lee S, Han S, Lee YJ, Kim JB, Seo EK, Jung CH. Triterpenoids from the Leaves of *Centella asiatica* Inhibit Ionizing Radiation-Induced Migration and Invasion of Human Lung Cancer Cells. Evid Based Complement Alternat Med. 2020 Sep 15;2020:3683460. doi: 10.1155/2020/3683460. PMID: 33029164; PMCID: PMC7532382.

Naidoo DB, Chuturgoon AA, Phulukdaree A, Guruprasad KP, Satyamoorthy K, Sewram V. Centella asiatica modulates cancer cachexia associated inflammatory cytokines and cell death in leukaemic THP-1 cells and peripheral blood mononuclear cells (PBMC's). BMC Complement Altern Med. 2017 Aug 1;17(1):377. doi: 10.1186/s12906-017-1865-2. PMID: 28764778; PMCID: PMC5540453.

Naidoo DB, Phulukdaree A, Krishnan A, Chuturgoon AA, Sewram V. *Centella asiatica* Modulates *Nrf-2* Antioxidant Mechanisms and Enhances Reactive Oxygen Species-Mediated Apoptotic Cell Death in Leukemic (THP-1) Cells. J Med Food. 2022 Jul;25(7):760-769. doi: 10.1089/jmf.2021.0173. Epub 2022 Jun 8. PMID: 35675643.

**Graviola (Annona muricata)**- Graviola fruit, stems, and leaves contain alkaloids, phenols, and acetogenins among other molecules. Acetogenins help selectively kill cancer cells by blocking their mitochondria's ability to create ATP. This then triggers the apoptosis process and cell death. This herb needs to be taken under the guidance of a knowledgeable holistic physician or herbalist as an overdose can cause nerve damage or Parkinson's-like symptoms.

Ilango S, Sahoo DK, Paital B, Kathirvel K, Gabriel JI, Subramaniam K, Jayachandran P, Dash RK, Hati AK, Behera TR, Mishra P, Nirmaladevi R. A Review on *Annona muricata* and Its Anticancer Activity. Cancers (Basel). 2022 Sep 19;14(18):4539. doi: 10.3390/cancers14184539. PMID: 36139697; PMCID: PMC9497149.

Qazi AK, Siddiqui JA, Jahan R, Chaudhary S, Walker LA, Sayed Z, Jones DT, Batra SK, Macha MA. Emerging therapeutic potential of graviola and its constituents in cancers. Carcinogenesis. 2018 Apr 5;39(4):522-533. doi: 10.1093/carcin/bgy024. PMID: 29462271; PMCID: PMC5888937.

Rojas-Armas JP, Arroyo-Acevedo JL, Palomino-Pacheco M, Ortiz-Sánchez JM, Calva J, Justil-Guerrero HJ, Castro-Luna A, Ramos-Cevallos N, Cieza-Macedo EC, Herrera-Calderon O. Phytochemical Constituents and Ameliorative Effect of the Essential Oil from *Annona muricata* L. Leaves in a Murine Model of Breast Cancer. Molecules. 2022 Mar 10;27(6):1818. doi: 10.3390/molecules27061818. PMID: 35335182; PMCID: PMC8949400.

-L-

**Larch (Larix spp.)**- This tree extract often comes in the form of a white fluffy powder. It is commonly sold under the name "Ara-6". Larch contains a molecule called Arabinogalactan that has been shown to stimulate natural killer (NK) cells and other cytokines that strengthen the immune system's ability to fight cancer. It is also a source of dietary fiber that nourishes the gut microbiome, and has been shown to increase the production of short-chain fatty acids such as butyrate and propionate that may have anticancer effects of their own.

Koizumi S, Masuko K, Wakita D, Tanaka S, Mitamura R, Kato Y, Tabata H, Nakahara M, Kitamura H, Nishimura T. Extracts of Larix Leptolepis effectively augments the generation of tumor antigen-specific cytotoxic T lymphocytes via activation of dendritic cells in TLR-2 and TLR-4-dependent manner. Cell Immunol. 2012 Mar-Apr;276(1-2):153-61. doi: 10.1016/j.cellimm.2012.05.002. Epub 2012 May 17. PMID: 22677561.

Hauer J, Anderer FA. Mechanism of stimulation of human natural killer cytotoxicity by arabinogalactan from Larix occidentalis. Cancer Immunol Immunother. 1993;36(4):237-44. doi: 10.1007/BF01740905. PMID: 8439987.

Tang S, Wang T, Huang C, Lai C, Fan Y, Yong Q. Sulfated modification of arabinogalactans from Larix principis-rupprechtii and their antitumor activities. Carbohydr Polym. 2019 Jul 1;215:207-212. doi: 10.1016/j.carbpol.2019.03.069. Epub 2019 Mar 21. PMID: 30981347.

**Lemon Balm (Melissa officinalis)**- This calming, soothing, and uplifting member of the mint family has a delicious lemon smell when the fresh leaves are crushed. Lemon Balm tea has been shown to help induce apoptosis and slow cancer-cell growth.

Kuo TT, Chang HY, Chen TY, Liu BC, Chen HY, Hsiung YC, Hsia SM, Chang CJ, Huang TC. *Melissa officinalis* Extract Induces Apoptosis and Inhibits Migration in Human Colorectal Cancer Cells. ACS Omega. 2020 Dec 3;5(49):31792-31800. doi: 10.1021/acsomega.0c04489. Erratum in: ACS Omega. 2021 Feb 18;6(8):6030. PMID: 33344833; PMCID: PMC7745433.

Kuo TT, Lin LC, Chang HY, Chiang PJ, Wu HY, Chen TY, Hsia SM, Huang TC. Quantitative Proteome Analysis Reveals Melissa officinalis Extract Targets Mitochondrial Respiration in Colon Cancer Cells. Molecules. 2022 Jul 15;27(14):4533. doi: 10.3390/molecules27144533. PMID: 35889404; PMCID: PMC9316399.\

Magalhães DB , Castro I , Lopes-Rodrigues V , Pereira JM , Barros L , Ferreira ICFR , Xavier CPR , Vasconcelos MH . Melissa officinalis L. ethanolic extract inhibits the growth of a lung cancer cell line by interfering with the cell cycle and inducing apoptosis. Food Funct. 2018 Jun 20;9(6):3134-3142. doi: 10.1039/c8fo00446c. PMID: 29790547.

**Licorice (Glycyrrhiza glabra)**- Is a major herb in Chinese and Western Herbal Medicine. It has anti-inflammatory, anti-tumor, anti-viral, and immune-enhancing effects. It has the power to increase NK cell activity and interferon production. It also supports the adrenal glands and can increase aldosterone, DHEA, and cortisol when they are out of balance. Licorice extract has also been shown helpful for reducing the side effects of chemo and radiation treatments.

Wang KL, Yu YC, Chen HY, Chiang YF, Ali M, Shieh TM, Hsia SM. Recent Advances in *Glycyrrhiza glabra* (Licorice)-Containing Herbs Alleviating Radiotherapy- and Chemotherapy-Induced Adverse Reactions in Cancer Treatment. Metabolites. 2022 Jun 9;12(6):535. doi: 10.3390/metabo12060535. PMID: 35736467; PMCID: PMC9227067.

Gioti K, Papachristodoulou A, Benaki D, Beloukas A, Vontzalidou A, Aligiannis N, Skaltsounis AL, Mikros E, Tenta R. *Glycyrrhiza glabra*-Enhanced Extract and Adriamycin Antiproliferative Effect on PC-3 Prostate Cancer Cells. Nutr Cancer. 2020;72(2):320-332. doi: 10.1080/01635581.2019.1632357. Epub 2019 Jul 5. PMID: 31274029.

Wang KL, Yu YC, Hsia SM. Perspectives on the Role of Isoliquiritigenin in Cancer. Cancers (Basel). 2021 Jan 1;13(1):115. doi: 10.3390/cancers13010115. PMID: 33401375; PMCID: PMC7795842.

-M-

**Magnolia (Magnolia grandiflora)**- The Magnolia tree, known for its large beautiful flowers, also contains anticancer molecules such as Honokiol and Magnolol. Research has shown that Honokiol works through ferroptosis, or iron-dependent cancer cell death.

Ranaware AM, Banik K, Deshpande V, Padmavathi G, Roy NK, Sethi G, Fan L, Kumar AP, Kunnumakkara AB. Magnolol: A Neolignan from the Magnolia Family for the Prevention and Treatment of Cancer. Int J Mol Sci. 2018 Aug 10;19(8):2362. doi: 10.3390/ijms19082362. PMID: 30103472; PMCID: PMC6121321.

Ma H, Bai X, Sun X, Li B, Zhu M, Dai Y, Huo Q, Li HM, Wu CZ. Anti-cancer effects of methanol-ethyl acetate partitioned fraction from Magnolia grandiflora in human non-small cell lung cancer H1975 cells. J Bioenerg Biomembr. 2020 Jun;52(3):175-183. doi: 10.1007/s10863-020-09828-6. Epub 2020 Apr 15. PMID: 32291605.

Guo C, Liu P, Deng G, Han Y, Chen Y, Cai C, Shen H, Deng G, Zeng S. Honokiol induces ferroptosis in colon cancer cells by regulating GPX4 activity. Am J Cancer Res. 2021 Jun 15;11(6):3039-3054. PMID: 34249443; PMCID: PMC8263670. come

**Maral Root (Raponticum carthamoides)**- Cancer specialist- herbalist Donnie Yance calls Raponticum, "the strongest anabolic (building up) agent in nature." It helps with bone building, and can help regenerate every organ in the body. It supports the prevention of weight loss and cachexia in advanced cancer, and it also has anticancer effects of its own.

Skała E, Synowiec E, Kowalczyk T, Śliwiński T, Sitarek P. *Rhaponticum carthamoides* Transformed Root Extract Has Potent Anticancer Activity in Human Leukemia and Lung Adenocarcinoma Cell Lines. Oxid Med Cell Longev. 2018 Dec 9;2018:8198652. doi: 10.1155/2018/8198652. PMID: 30622675; PMCID: PMC6304841.

Skała E, Sitarek P, Toma M, Szemraj J, Radek M, Nieborowska-Skorska M, Skorski T, Wysokińska H, Śliwiński T. Inhibition of human glioma cell proliferation by altered Bax/Bcl-2-p53 expression and apoptosis induction by Rhaponticum carthamoides extracts from transformed and normal roots. J Pharm Pharmacol. 2016 Nov;68(11):1454-1464. doi: 10.1111/jphp.12619. Epub 2016 Oct 2. PMID: 27696406.

Skała E, Kowalczyk T, Toma M, Szemraj J, Radek M, Pytel D, Wieczfinska J, Wysokińska H, Śliwiński T, Sitarek P. Induction of apoptosis in human glioma cell lines of various grades through the ROS-mediated mitochondrial pathway and caspase activation by Rhaponticum carthamoides transformed root extract. Mol Cell Biochem. 2018 Aug;445(1-2):89-97. doi: 10.1007/s11010-017-3254-z. Epub 2017 Dec 14. PMID: 29238899.

**Marijuana / Hemp (Cannabis sativa or indica)**- Medical marijuana has been studied for many decades and has over 35,000 scientific articles in the Pubmed database describing the effects of cannabis on cancer. Molecules from the cannabis plant are called cannabinoids and include abbreviations like: THC, CBD, CBDA, and CBC. Most of these molecules have been found to have anticancer effects. In addition, Cannabis contains various terpenes that are the tiny molecules also found in essential oils that include: Linalool, Myrcene, Limonene, Caryophyllene, and more. These terpenes also have demonstrated anticancer effects so cannabis is a symphony of healing molecules. THC is the main psychoactive molecule that causes a "high", and is why cannabis is still illegal at the federal level in the United States. Hemp extracts are the legal versions that contain next to no THC, but still have many of the other anticancer cannabinoids and terpenes, so it is not necessarily required to get high, break the law, or obtain a medical marijuana card in order to receive the benefits of cannabis for cancer. At the time of this writing, 38 U.S. States have legalized medical marijuana programs. Cancer is recognized as one of the approved conditions for medical marijuana because it has demonstrated anti-cancer effects, and it also helps to increase appetite and reduce nausea and vomiting caused by conventional chemotherapy treatments. Direct anticancer effects of cannabis include: decreased tumor-cell proliferation, slowed tumor invasion and metastasis, reduced angiogenesis and chemoresistance, as well as induction of apoptosis and autophagy (forms of cell death). If you do not want the psychoactive effects of THC or live in an area where legal medical marijuana is not available you can look for cannabis essential oil that will include many of the anti-cancer terpene molecules as well as full spectrum hemp paste that includes all of the legal cannabinoids that still have powerful anti-cancer properties.

**Pellati F, Borgonetti V, Brighenti V, Biagi M, Benvenuti S, Corsi L.** *Cannabis sativa* L. and Nonpsychoactive Cannabinoids: Their Chemistry and Role against Oxidative Stress, Inflammation, and Cancer. Biomed Res Int. 2018 Dec 4;2018:1691428. doi: 10.1155/2018/1691428. PMID: 30627539; PMCID: PMC6304621.

ElSohly MA, Radwan MM, Gul W, Chandra S, Galal A. Phytochemistry of Cannabis sativa L. Prog Chem Org Nat Prod. 2017;103:1-36. doi: 10.1007/978-3-319-45541-9_1. PMID: 28120229.

Abrams DI. Cannabis, Cannabinoids and Cannabis-Based Medicines in Cancer Care. Integr Cancer Ther. 2022 Jan-Dec;21:15347354221081772. doi: 10.1177/15347354221081772. PMID: 35225051; PMCID: PMC8882944.

**Milk thistle (Silybum marianum)**- The seeds of Milk Thistle are especially helpful for hepatitis and liver cancer. This herb protects the liver from toxic effects of chemo and radiation. It helps certain chemotherapies such as Cisplatin and Doxorubicin work better against killing cancer cells.

Emadi SA, Ghasemzadeh Rahbardar M, Mehri S, Hosseinzadeh H. A review of therapeutic potentials of milk thistle (*Silybum marianum* L.) and its main constituent, silymarin, on cancer, and their related patents. Iran J Basic Med Sci. 2022 Oct;25(10):1166-1176. doi: 10.22038/IJBMS.2022.63200.13961. PMID: 36311193; PMCID: PMC9588316.

Yassin NYS, AbouZid SF, El-Kalaawy AM, Ali TM, Almehmadi MM, Ahmed OM. Silybum marianum total extract, silymarin and silibinin abate hepatocarcinogenesis and hepatocellular carcinoma growth via modulation of the HGF/c-Met, Wnt/β-catenin, and PI3K/Akt/mTOR signaling pathways. Biomed Pharmacother. 2022 Jan;145:112409. doi: 10.1016/j.biopha.2021.112409. Epub 2021 Nov 12. PMID: 34781148.

Fallah M, Davoodvandi A, Nikmanzar S, Aghili S, Mirazimi SMA, Aschner M, Rashidian A, Hamblin MR, Chamanara M, Naghsh N, Mirzaei H. Silymarin (milk thistle extract) as a therapeutic agent in gastrointestinal cancer. Biomed Pharmacother. 2021 Oct;142:112024. doi: 10.1016/j.biopha.2021.112024. Epub 2021 Aug 13. PMID: 34399200; PMCID: PMC8458260.

**Mistletoe (Viscum album)**- As an injectable, this medicine is one of the most used complementary cancer therapies in Europe, often under the brand names of Iscador or Helixor. It is tumor inhibiting, enhances NK cells, increases depleted white cell counts after chemo or radiation, and contains selectively cancer-toxic peptides. It is also available in Gemmotherapy (plant bud extract) and homeopathic forms.

Pelzer F, Loef M, Martin DD, Baumgartner S. Cancer-related fatigue in patients treated with mistletoe extracts: a systematic review and meta-analysis. Support Care Cancer. 2022 Aug;30(8):6405-6418. doi: 10.1007/s00520-022-06921-x. Epub 2022 Mar 3. PMID: 35239008; PMCID: PMC9213316.

Nazaruk J, Orlikowski P. Phytochemical profile and therapeutic potential of Viscum album L. Nat Prod Res. 2016;30(4):373-85. doi: 10.1080/14786419.2015.1022776. Epub 2015 Mar 27. PMID: 25813519.

Rostock M. Die Misteltherapie in der Behandlung von Patienten mit einer Krebserkrankung [Mistletoe in the treatment of cancer patients]. Bundesgesundheitsblatt Gesundheitsforschung Gesundheitsschutz. 2020 May;63(5):535-540. German. doi: 10.1007/s00103-020-03122-x. PMID: 32211937.

**Moringa (Moringa oleifera)**- This tree is currently used as a superfood around the world. It has nutritive, detoxifying, and blood-glucose balancing effects that make it a great support herb during cancer treatment. This nutrient powerhouse has also shown direct anticancer effects in some lab studies.

Wu YY, Xu YM, Lau ATY. Anti-Cancer and Medicinal Potentials of Moringa Isothiocyanate. Molecules. 2021 Dec 11;26(24):7512. doi: 10.3390/molecules26247512. PMID: 34946594; PMCID: PMC8708952.

Tiloke C, Anand K, Gengan RM, Chuturgoon AA. Moringa oleifera and their phytonanoparticles: Potential antiproliferative agents against cancer. Biomed Pharmacother. 2018 Dec;108:457-466. doi: 10.1016/j.biopha.2018.09.060. Epub 2018 Sep 18. PMID: 30241049.

Masarkar N, Ray SK, Saleem Z, Mukherjee S. Potential anti-cancer activity of Moringa oleifera derived bio-active compounds targeting hypoxia-inducible factor-1 alpha in breast cancer. J Complement Integr Med. 2023 Sep 18. doi: 10.1515/jcim-2023-0182. Epub ahead of print. PMID: 37712721.

**Mustard Seed (Sinapsis alba)**- In addition to its use as a food spice, mustard seed contains molecules called isothiocyanates that show antioxidant, apoptotic, and cancer growth-inhibiting effects. Mustard is commonly used to promote circulation, warming, digestion, and help with infections.

Boscaro V, Boffa L, Binello A, Amisano G, Fornasero S, Cravotto G, Gallicchio M. Antiproliferative, Proapoptotic, Antioxidant and Antimicrobial Effects of Sinapis nigra L. and Sinapis alba L. Extracts. Molecules. 2018 Nov 16;23(11):3004. doi: 10.3390/molecules23113004. PMID: 30453590; PMCID: PMC6278512.

Jurkowska H, Wróbel M, Szlęzak D, Jasek-Gajda E. New aspects of antiproliferative activity of 4-hydroxybenzyl isothiocyanate, a natural $H_2S$-donor. Amino Acids. 2018 Jun;50(6):699-709. doi: 10.1007/s00726-018-2546-2. Epub 2018 Mar 5. PMID: 29508061; PMCID: PMC5945766.

Lamy E, Garcia-Käufer M, Prinzhorn J, Mersch-Sundermann V. Antigenotoxic action of isothiocyanate-containing mustard as determined by two cancer biomarkers in a human intervention trial. Eur J Cancer Prev. 2012 Jul;21(4):400-6. doi: 10.1097/CEJ.0b013e32834ef140. PMID: 22157087.

**Myrrh (Commiphora myrrha)**- Famous as one of the three Christmas gifts of the wise men to the baby Jesus, this herb is traditionally used as an antiseptic and wound healer. Myrrh has been shown to increase the activity of macrophages, decrease inflammation, and increase the apoptosis of cancer cells.

Girisa S, Parama D, Harsha C, Banik K, Kunnumakkara AB. Potential of guggulsterone, a farnesoid X receptor antagonist, in the prevention and treatment of cancer. Explor Target Antitumor Ther. 2020;1(5):313-342. doi: 10.37349/etat.2020.00019. Epub 2020 Oct 30. PMID: 36046484; PMCID: PMC9400725.

Gao W, Su X, Dong X, Chen Y, Zhou C, Xin P, Yu C, Wei T. Cycloartan-24-ene-1α,2α,3β-triol, a cycloartane-type triterpenoid from the resinous exudates of Commiphora myrrha, induces apoptosis in human prostatic cancer PC-3 cells. Oncol Rep. 2015 Mar;33(3):1107-14. doi: 10.3892/or.2015.3725. Epub 2015 Jan 15. PMID: 25591732.

Suliman RS, Alghamdi SS, Ali R, Aljatli D, Aljammaz NA, Huwaizi S, Suliman R, Kahtani KM, Albadrani GM, Barhoumi T, Altolayyan A, Rahman I. The Role of Myrrh Metabolites in Cancer, Inflammation, and Wound Healing: Prospects for a Multi-Targeted Drug Therapy. Pharmaceuticals (Basel). 2022 Jul 29;15(8):944. doi: 10.3390/ph15080944. PMID: 36015092; PMCID: PMC9416713.

## -O-

**Oregon Grape (Mahonia aquifolium)-** This plant contains berberine that has proven anticancer properties and inhibits tumor growth through the activation of the AMPK pathway that slows cell growth and proliferation. Oregon Grape is also commonly used for stomach ulcers, GERD, digestive support, and to treat infections.

Andreicuţ AD, Fischer-Fodor E, Pârvu AE, Ţigu AB, Cenariu M, Pârvu M, Cătoi FA, Irimie A. Antitumoral and Immunomodulatory Effect of *Mahonia aquifolium* Extracts. Oxid Med Cell Longev. 2019 Dec 14;2019:6439021. doi: 10.1155/2019/6439021. PMID: 31949880; PMCID: PMC6948282.

Tuzimski T, Petruczynik A, Plech T, Kaproń B, Makuch-Kocka A, Szultka-Młyńska M, Misiurek J, Buszewski B, Waksmundzka-Hajnos M. Determination of Selected Isoquinoline Alkaloids from *Chelidonium majus*, *Mahonia aquifolium* and *Sanguinaria canadensis* Extracts by Liquid Chromatography and Their In Vitro and In Vivo Cytotoxic Activity against Human Cancer Cells. Int J Mol Sci. 2023 Mar 28;24(7):6360. doi: 10.3390/ijms24076360. PMID: 37047332; PMCID: PMC10093986.

Tuzimski T, Petruczynik A, Kaproń B, Makuch-Kocka A, Szultka-Młyńska M, Misiurek J, Szymczak G, Buszewski B. Determination of Cytotoxic Activity of Selected Isoquinoline Alkaloids and Plant Extracts Obtained from Various Parts of *Mahonia aquifolium* Collected in Various Vegetation Seasons. Molecules. 2021 Feb 4;26(4):816. doi: 10.3390/molecules26040816. PMID: 33557343; PMCID: PMC7915140.

## -P-

**Pao Pereira (Geissospermum vellosii)-** An Amazon Rainforest herb that stopped cancer cell proliferation without affecting healthy cells. It shows anticancer effects on a large range of human cancers. It can induce apoptosis and cell cycle arrest with no known side effects. It helps reduce PSA and BPH in men. It has also been shown to help chemotherapy work better.

(Natural Source International- https://www.maisonbeljanski.com)

Li JM, Huang YC, Kuo YH, Cheng CC, Kuan FC, Chang SF, Lee YR, Chin CC, Shi CS. Flavopereirine Suppresses the Growth of Colorectal Cancer Cells through P53 Signaling Dependence. Cancers (Basel). 2019 Jul 22;11(7):1034. doi: 10.3390/cancers11071034. PMID: 31336690; PMCID: PMC6678721.

Yu J, Chen Q. The plant extract of Pao pereira potentiates carboplatin effects against ovarian cancer. Pharm Biol. 2014 Jan;52(1):36-43. doi: 10.3109/13880209.2013.808232. Epub 2013 Sep 13. PMID: 24033267.

Bemis DL, Capodice JL, Desai M, Katz AE, Buttyan R. beta-carboline alkaloid-enriched extract from the amazonian rain forest tree pao pereira suppresses prostate cancer cells. J Soc Integr Oncol. 2009 Spring;7(2):59-65. PMID: 19476740; PMCID: PMC6358020.

**Pao Tariri (Quassia amara)**- Is an herb from the South-American Amazon. According to the research of Mirko Beljanski, this herb synergizes well with Pao Pereira, and is available in a combined formula called PAO V "FM" from the site below.

(Natural Source International-https://www.maisonbeljanski.com)

Robert G, Jullian V, Jacquel A, Ginet C, Dufies M, Torino S, Pottier A, Peyrade F, Tartare-Deckert S, Bourdy G, Deharo E, Auberger P. Simalikalactone E (SkE), a new weapon in the armamentarium of drugs targeting cancers that exhibit constitutive activation of the ERK pathway. Oncotarget. 2012 Dec;3(12):1688-99. doi: 10.18632/oncotarget.791. PMID: 23518796; PMCID: PMC3681504.

Bourdy G, Aubertin C, Jullian V, Deharo E. Quassia "biopiracy" case and the Nagoya Protocol: A researcher's perspective. J Ethnopharmacol. 2017 Jul 12;206:290-297. doi: 10.1016/j.jep.2017.05.030. Epub 2017 May 31. PMID: 28576580.

**Pau d' Arco (Tabebuia avellanedae)**- This South American plant, also known as Lapacho, produces molecules called lapachol, lapachone, and naphthoquinone which weaken and suppress tumor formation. It has mild pain relieving properties and it is traditionally used as an antifungal antibacterial and antiparasitic.

Telang N, Nair HB, Wong GYC. Growth inhibitory efficacy and anti-aromatase activity of *Tabebuia avellanedae* in a model for post-menopausal Luminal A breast cancer. Biomed Rep. 2019 Nov;11(5):222-229. doi: 10.3892/br.2019.1244. Epub 2019 Oct 3. PMID: 31632670; PMCID: PMC6792322.

Yamashita M, Kaneko M, Iida A, Tokuda H, Nishimura K. Stereoselective synthesis and cytotoxicity of a cancer chemopreventive naphthoquinone from Tabebuia avellanedae. Bioorg Med Chem Lett. 2007 Dec 1;17(23):6417-20. doi: 10.1016/j.bmcl.2007.10.005. Epub 2007 Oct 5. PMID: 17950604.

Queiroz ML, Valadares MC, Torello CO, Ramos AL, Oliveira AB, Rocha FD, Arruda VA, Accorci WR. Comparative studies of the effects of Tabebuia avellanedae bark extract and beta-lapachone on the hematopoietic response of tumour-bearing mice. J Ethnopharmacol. 2008 May 8;117(2):228-35. doi: 10.1016/j.jep.2008.01.034. Epub 2008 Feb 8. PMID: 18343063.

**Paw paw (Asimina triloba)**- Dr. Jerry McLaughlin of Purdue University has been one of the most prominent researchers of Paw Paw. It contains molecules called acetogenins that block cancer cell's ability to make ATP for energy. This starves the cancer cells of needed fuel, which then die. The twigs of the Paw Paw tree contain the highest amounts of acetogenins.

Paw Paw can also help reduce multidrug resistance in cancer cells. Nature's Sunshine sells a Paw Paw extract with the highest reputation. This should not be used long-term or as a preventative for cancer, but only when active cancer is present.

https://www.naturessunshine.com/product/paw-paw/

Nam JS, Park SY, Lee SO, Lee HJ, Jang HL, Rhee YH. The growth-inhibitory effects of pawpaw (Asimina triloba [L.] Dunal) roots, twigs, leaves, and fruit against human gastric (AGS) and cervical (HeLa) cancer cells and their anti-inflammatory activities. Mol Biol Rep. 2021 Mar;48(3):2173-2181. doi: 10.1007/s11033-021-06226-y. Epub 2021 Feb 25. PMID: 33630206.

McLaughlin JL. Paw paw and cancer: annonaceous acetogenins from discovery to commercial products. J Nat Prod. 2008 Jul;71(7):1311-21. doi: 10.1021/np800191t. Epub 2008 Jul 4. PMID: 18598079.

Zhao GX, Miesbauer LR, Smith DL, McLaughlin JL. Asimin, asiminacin, and asiminecin: novel highly cytotoxic asimicin isomers from Asimina triloba. J Med Chem. 1994 Jun 24;37(13):1971-6. doi: 10.1021/jm00039a009. PMID: 8027979.

**Plantain (Plantago major)**- This herb is a common first aid for insect bites and poison ivy. It contains flavonoids that are able to strongly inhibit the proliferation of multiple cancer-cell lines. Plantain is also used as a treatment for oral mucositis from radiation therapy for head and neck cancer.

Kartini, Piyaviriyakul S, Thongpraditchote S, Siripong P, Vallisuta O. Effects of *Plantago major* Extracts and Its Chemical Compounds on Proliferation of Cancer Cells and Cytokines Production of Lipopolysaccharide-activated THP-1 Macrophages. Pharmacogn Mag. 2017 Jul-Sep;13(51):393-399. doi: 10.4103/pm.pm_406_16. Epub 2017 Jul 19. PMID: 28839362; PMCID: PMC5551355.

Soltani GM, Hemati S, Sarvizadeh M, Kamalinejad M, Tafazoli V, Latifi SA. Efficacy of the plantago major L. syrup on radiation induced oral mucositis in head and neck cancer patients: A randomized, double blind, placebo-controlled clinical trial. Complement Ther Med. 2020 Jun;51:102397. doi: 10.1016/j.ctim.2020.102397. Epub 2020 Apr 30. PMID: 32507421.

Cabrera-Jaime S, Martínez C, Ferro-García T, Giner-Boya P, Icart-Isern T, Estrada-Masllorens JM, Fernández-Ortega P. Efficacy of Plantago major, chlorhexidine 0.12% and sodium bicarbonate 5% solution in the treatment of oral mucositis in cancer patients with solid tumour: A feasibility randomised triple-blind phase III clinical trial. Eur J Oncol Nurs. 2018 Feb;32:40-47. doi: 10.1016/j.ejon.2017.11.006. Epub 2017 Dec 14. PMID: 29353631.

Gálvez M, Martín-Cordero C, López-Lázaro M, Cortés F, Ayuso MJ. Cytotoxic effect of Plantago spp. on cancer cell lines. J Ethnopharmacol. 2003 Oct;88(2-3):125-30. doi: 10.1016/s0378-8741(03)00192-2. PMID: 12963131.

-R-

**Red Clover (Trifolium pratense)**- Is one of the main ingredients in the Hoxey formula, the Eclectic Trifolium compound, and Dr Chrstopher's Red Clover Combination Tea. It is considered a cleanser and blood purifier in herbal traditions. It has anti-angiogenic, anti-estrogenic, and anti-cancer properties. It has been used most often in melanomas, and breast, prostate, and colon cancers.

Fritz H, Seely D, Flower G, Skidmore B, Fernandes R, Vadeboncoeur S, Kennedy D, Cooley K, Wong R, Sagar S, Sabri E, Fergusson D. Soy, red clover, and isoflavones and breast cancer: a systematic review. PLoS One. 2013 Nov 28;8(11):e81968. doi: 10.1371/journal.pone.0081968. PMID: 24312387; PMCID: PMC3842968.

Akbaribazm M, Khazaei MR, Khazaei M. *Trifolium pratense* L. (red clover) extract and doxorubicin synergistically inhibits proliferation of 4T1 breast cancer in tumor-bearing BALB/c mice through modulation of apoptosis and increase antioxidant and anti-inflammatory related pathways. Food Sci Nutr. 2020 Jul 6;8(8):4276-4290. doi: 10.1002/fsn3.1724. PMID: 32884708; PMCID: PMC7455927.

Akbaribazm M, Khazaei MR, Khazaei F, Khazaei M. Doxorubicin and *Trifolium pratense* L. (Red clover) extract synergistically inhibits brain and lung metastases in 4T1 tumor-bearing BALB/c mice. Food Sci Nutr. 2020 Sep 1;8(10):5557-5570. doi: 10.1002/fsn3.1820. PMID: 33133558; PMCID: PMC7590334.

-S-

**Saw Palmetto (Serenoa repens)**- Is most often used in prostate cancer and Benign prostate hyperplasia (BPH). It has molecules that block the 5-alpha reductase enzyme that converts testosterone to the more powerful dihydrotestosterone (DHT). It is often used in combination with other herbs for synergistic hormonal effects.

Baron A, Mancini M, Caldwell E, Cabrelle A, Bernardi P, Pagano F. Serenoa repens extract targets mitochondria and activates the intrinsic apoptotic pathway in human prostate cancer cells. BJU Int. 2009 May;103(9):1275-83. doi: 10.1111/j.1464-410X.2008.08266.x. Epub 2009 Jan 14. PMID: 19154468.

Che Y, Hou S, Kang Z, Lin Q. Serenoa repens induces growth arrest and apoptosis of human multiple myeloma cells via inactivation of STAT 3 signaling. Oncol Rep. 2009 Aug;22(2):377-83. PMID: 19578780.

Habib FK, Ross M, Ho CK, Lyons V, Chapman K. Serenoa repens (Permixon) inhibits the 5alpha-reductase activity of human prostate cancer cell lines without interfering with PSA expression. Int J Cancer. 2005 Mar 20;114(2):190-4. doi: 10.1002/ijc.20701. PMID: 15543614.

**Self Heal (Prunella vulgaris)** - Also called "Heal All", this herb has been used at high doses of 30g per day for cancer. It can help shrink tumors, and has been most studied in breast cancer. In traditional herbalism it has been used for dizziness, coughs, dermatitis, sore throats, and wounds.

Zhang X, Shen T, Zhou X, Tang X, Gao R, Xu L, Wang L, Zhou Z, Lin J, Hu Y. Network pharmacology based virtual screening of active constituents of Prunella vulgaris L. and the molecular mechanism against breast cancer. Sci Rep. 2020 Sep 25;10(1):15730. doi: 10.1038/s41598-020-72797-8. PMID: 32978480; PMCID: PMC7519149.

Luo H, Zhao L, Li Y, Xia B, Lin Y, Xie J, Wu P, Liao D, Zhang Z, Lin L. An *in vivo* and *in vitro* assessment of the anti-breast cancer activity of crude extract and fractions from *Prunella vulgaris* L. Heliyon. 2022 Oct 19;8(11):e11183. doi: 10.1016/j.heliyon.2022.e11183. PMID: 36345524; PMCID: PMC9636486.

Yu F, Zhang L, Ma R, Liu C, Wang Q, Yin D. The Antitumour Effect of *Prunella vulgaris* Extract on Thyroid Cancer Cells In Vitro and In Vivo. Evid Based Complement Alternat Med. 2021 Jan 8;2021:8869323. doi: 10.1155/2021/8869323. PMID: 33505511; PMCID: PMC7811421.

**Sheep Sorrel (Rumex acetosella)**- This is one of the original herbs in the Essiac tea cancer formula. Though little scientific research is available for this specific species, many of the Rumex family of plants have been studied for their anti-cancer properties due to their flavonoid and anthraquinone content.

Kim HY, Seo JE, Lee H, Bae CH, Ha KT, Kim S. *Rumex japonicus* Houtt. Extract Suppresses Colitis-Associated Colorectal Cancer by Regulating Inflammation and Tight-Junction Integrity in Mice. Front Pharmacol. 2022 Jul 5;13:946909. doi: 10.3389/fphar.2022.946909. PMID: 35865942; PMCID: PMC9294457.

Riffat B, Ejaz A, Hina S, Javed I, Saira T, Tariq M. Rumex dentatus could be a potent alternative to treatment of microbial infections and of breast cancer. J Tradit Chin Med. 2019 Dec;39(6):772-779. PMID: 32186147.

Ginovyan M, Javrushyan H, Petrosyan G, Kusznierewicz B, Koss-Mikołajczyk I, Koziara Z, Kuczyńska M, Jakubek P, Karapetyan A, Sahakyan N, Maloyan A, Bartoszek A, Avtandilyan N. Anti-cancer effect of Rumex obtusifolius in combination with arginase/nitric oxide synthase inhibitors via downregulation of oxidative stress, inflammation, and polyamine synthesis. Int J Biochem Cell Biol. 2023 May;158:106396. doi: 10.1016/j.biocel.2023.106396. Epub 2023 Mar 12. PMID: 36918141.

**Slippery Elm (Ulmus rubra)**- This common tree bark has powerful tissue healing effects, and due to its slippery mucilaginous nature, can coat and soothe tissue damage from radiation and chemotherapy. This can be done internally for the GI tract or externally as a poultice on radiation burns.

Many species of elm have been studied for their ability to slow cancer-cell growth and kill cancer cells through apoptosis and autophagy.

Hong SO, Choi IK, Jeong W, Lee SR, Sung HJ, Hong SS, Seo JH. Ulmus davidiana Nakai induces apoptosis and autophagy on non-small cell lung cancer cells. J Ethnopharmacol. 2017 Apr 18;202:1-11. doi: 10.1016/j.jep.2017.03.009. Epub 2017 Mar 9. PMID: 28284790.

Ahn J, Lee JS, Yang KM. Ultrafine particles of Ulmus davidiana var. japonica induce apoptosis of gastric cancer cells via activation of caspase and endoplasmic reticulum stress. Arch Pharm Res. 2014 Jun;37(6):783-92. doi: 10.1007/s12272-013-0312-2. Epub 2014 Jan 7. PMID: 24395528; PMCID: PMC4047481.

Ren Y, Qin Z, Wang Z, Wei S, Chen H, Zhu T, Liu L, Zhao Y, Ding B, Song W. Condensed tannins from Ulmus pumila L. leaves induce G2/M phase arrest and apoptosis via caspase-cascade activation in TFK-1 cholangiocarcinoma cells. J Food Biochem. 2022 Oct;46(10):e14374. doi: 10.1111/jfbc.14374. Epub 2022 Aug 20. PMID: 35986624.

**Suma (Pfaffia paniculata)**- Suma, also known as Brazilian ginseng, is revered for its adaptogenic properties and belongs to a group of herbs called adaptogens. Adaptogens are recognized for their ability to help the body adapt to various internal and external stressors, ranging from illness and sleep deprivation to excessive workload. These herbs aim to enhance both physical and mental performance, endurance, and overall vitality.
Suma, specifically, possesses adaptogenic qualities that stimulate the immune response. It is believed to contribute to the healing and recovery process, particularly in cases of chronic illnesses such as cancer and diabetes. It has been demonstrated in scientific studies that Suma is toxic to cancer cells and reduces the angiogenesis process.

Rahamouz-Haghighi S, Sharafi A. Antiproliferative assay of suma or Brazilian ginseng (*Hebanthe eriantha*) methanolic extract on HCT116 and 4T1 cancer cell lines, *in vitro* toxicity on *Artemia salina* larvae, and antibacterial activity. Nat Prod Res. 2023 Jun 19:1-5. doi: 10.1080/14786419.2023.2225688. Epub ahead of print. PMID: 37337697.

Nagamine MK, da Silva TC, Matsuzaki P, Pinello KC, Cogliati B, Pizzo CR, Akisue G, Haraguchi M, Górniak SL, Sinhorini IL, Rao KV, Barbuto JA, Dagli ML. Cytotoxic effects of butanolic extract from Pfaffia paniculata (Brazilian ginseng) on cultured human breast cancer cell line MCF-7. Exp Toxicol Pathol. 2009 Jan;61(1):75-82. doi: 10.1016/j.etp.2008.01.017. Epub 2008 May 16. PMID: 18485683.

Carneiro CS, Costa-Pinto FA, da Silva AP, Pinello KC, da Silva TC, Matsuzaki P, Nagamine MK, Górniak SL, Haraguchi M, Akisue G, Dagli ML. Pfaffia paniculata (Brazilian ginseng) methanolic extract reduces angiogenesis in mice. Exp Toxicol Pathol. 2007 Aug;58(6):427-31. doi: 10.1016/j.etp.2006.11.005. Epub 2007 May 3. PMID: 17481871.

**Sundew (Drosera rotundifolia)**- Has similar active anticancer molecules as Venus Fly Trap, but is more affordable. It is a non-toxic treatment for many cancer types, and it is used traditionally for all types of coughs. Studies have shown some anti-inflammatory properties as well as the ability to induce apoptosis and cell cycle arrest in cancer cells.

Li S, Chen N, Gaddes ER, Zhang X, Dong C, Wang Y. A Drosera-bioinspired hydrogel for catching and killing cancer cells. Sci Rep. 2015 Sep 23;5:14297. doi: 10.1038/srep14297. PMID: 26396063; PMCID: PMC4585793.

Ghate NB, Das A, Chaudhuri D, Panja S, Mandal N. Sundew plant, a potential source of anti-inflammatory agents, selectively induces G2/M arrest and apoptosis in MCF-7 cells through upregulation of p53 and Bax/Bcl-2 ratio. Cell Death Discov. 2016 Jan 18;2:15062. doi: 10.1038/cddiscovery.2015.62. PMID: 27551490; PMCID: PMC4979533.

Toton E, Kedziora I, Romaniuk-Drapala A, Konieczna N, Kaczmarek M, Lisiak N, Paszel-Jaworska A, Rybska A, Duszynska W, Budzianowski J, Rybczynska M, Rubis B. Effect of 3-O-acetylaleuritolic acid from in vitro-cultured Drosera spatulata on cancer cells survival and migration. Pharmacol Rep. 2020 Feb;72(1):166-178. doi: 10.1007/s43440-019-00008-x. Epub 2020 Jan 10. PMID: 32016855.

**Sweet Annie- (Artemisia annua)**- Contains a flavonoid called Artemisinin that reacts with Iron to create free-radical damage to cancer cells. It has been found to be effective at killing breast cancer cells. This herb family is also used for malaria in areas of the world where it is prevalent.

Efferth T. From ancient herb to modern drug: Artemisia annua and artemisinin for cancer therapy. Semin Cancer Biol. 2017 Oct;46:65-83. doi: 10.1016/j.semcancer.2017.02.009. Epub 2017 Feb 28. PMID: 28254675.

Hu Y, Guo N, Yang T, Yan J, Wang W, Li X. The Potential Mechanisms by which Artemisinin and Its Derivatives Induce Ferroptosis in the Treatment of Cancer. Oxid Med Cell Longev. 2022 Jan 4;2022:1458143. doi: 10.1155/2022/1458143. PMID: 35028002; PMCID: PMC8752222.

Dawood H, Celik I, Ibrahim RS. Computational biology and in vitro studies for anticipating cancer-related molecular targets of sweet wormwood (Artemisia annua). BMC Complement Med Ther. 2023 Sep 8;23(1):312. doi: 10.1186/s12906-023-04135-0. PMID: 37684586; PMCID: PMC10492370.

-T-

**Tulsi (Ocimum sanctum)**- Also known as Holy Basil, this popular Ayurvedic herb has been shown to have anti inflammatory, pain-relieving, antidiabetic, liver protective, hypolipidemic, antistress, and immunomodulatory properties. Its molecules including: eugenol, rosmarinic acid, apigenin, luteolin, β-sitosterol, and carnosic acid have all shown anticancer effects.

Baliga MS, Jimmy R, Thilakchand KR, Sunitha V, Bhat NR, Saldanha E, Rao S, Rao P, Arora R, Palatty PL. Ocimum sanctum L (Holy Basil or Tulsi) and its phytochemicals in the prevention and treatment of cancer. Nutr Cancer. 2013;65 Suppl 1:26-35. doi: 10.1080/01635581.2013.785010. PMID: 23682780.

Bhattacharyya P, Bishayee A. Ocimum sanctum Linn. (Tulsi): an ethnomedicinal plant for the prevention and treatment of cancer. Anticancer Drugs. 2013 Aug;24(7):659-66. doi: 10.1097/CAD.0b013e328361aca1. PMID: 23629478.

Jiang H, Sathiyavimal S, Cai L, Devanesan S, Sayed SRM, Jhanani GK, Lin J. Tulsi (Ocimum sanctum) mediated Co nanoparticles with their anti-inflammatory, anti-cancer, and methyl orange dye adsorption properties. Environ Res. 2023 Nov 1;236(Pt 2):116749. doi: 10.1016/j.envres.2023.116749. Epub 2023 Jul 27. PMID: 37507040.

-W-

**Wormwood (Artemisia absinthium)-** This herb is commonly used for parasites and was a main ingredient that made the infamous absinthe drink that was popular in the late 19th and early 20th centuries. It contains a flavonoid called Artemisinin that reacts with Iron to create free radical damage to cancer cells. Has been found to be effective at killing breast cancer cells.

Efferth T. From ancient herb to modern drug: Artemisia annua and artemisinin for cancer therapy. Semin Cancer Biol. 2017 Oct;46:65-83. doi: 10.1016/j.semcancer.2017.02.009. Epub 2017 Feb 28. PMID: 28254675.

Slezakova S, Ruda-Kucerova J. Anticancer Activity of Artemisinin and its Derivatives. Anticancer Res. 2017 Nov;37(11):5995-6003. doi: 10.21873/anticanres.12046. PMID: 29061778.

Ali M, Iqbal R, Safdar M, Murtaza S, Mustafa G, Sajjad M, Bukhari SA, Huma T. Antioxidant and antibacterial activities of Artemisia absinthium and Citrus paradisi extracts repress viability of aggressive liver cancer cell line. Mol Biol Rep. 2021 Dec;48(12):7703-7710. doi: 10.1007/s11033-021-06777-0. Epub 2021 Nov 9. Erratum in: Mol Biol Rep. 2022 Apr;49(4):3367. PMID: 34755263.

-Y-

**Yellow dock (Rumex crispus)-** This herb is a classic ingredient in the Hoxsey Tea formula and Eli Jones' scrophularia compound. It contains the anthraquinone glycoside emodin and acts as a mild laxative and helps to nourish and detoxify the body. It has been shown to protect DNA from damage, reduce inflammation, and slow cancer cell growth.

Eom T, Kim E, Kim JS. In Vitro Antioxidant, Antiinflammation, and Anticancer Activities and Anthraquinone Content from *Rumex crispus* Root Extract and Fractions. Antioxidants (Basel). 2020 Aug 10;9(8):726. doi: 10.3390/antiox9080726. PMID: 32784977; PMCID: PMC7464605.

Shiwani S, Singh NK, Wang MH. Carbohydrase inhibition and anti-cancerous and free radical scavenging properties along with DNA and protein protection ability of methanolic root extracts of Rumex crispus. Nutr Res Pract. 2012 Oct;6(5):389-95. doi: 10.4162/nrp.2012.6.5.389. Epub 2012 Oct 31. PMID: 23198017; PMCID: PMC3506869.

## Traditional Cancer Formulas

**Hoxsey Formula-** Red Clover, Licorice Root, Poke Root, Barberry, Stillingia, Cascara Sagrada, Prickly Ash Bark, Burdock Root, Buckthorn Bark, Potassium iodide

**Dr Christopher's- Red Clover Combination-** Red Clover, Chaparral, Licorice Root, Poke Root, Peach Leaf, Oregon Grape Root, Stillingia, Cascara Sagrada Bark, Sarsaparilla Root, Prickly Ash Bark, Burdock Root, Buckthorn Bark.

**Professional Formulas- Hoxey-Like Formula-** Burdock, Red Clover, Oregon Grape, Poke, Queen's-Delight, Cascara Sagrada, Prickly-Ash, Wild Indigo, Licorice, Anise, Lugol's solution

**Eli Jones Scrophularia Compound-** Scrophularia, poke, rumex, false bittersweet, mayapple, juniper, corydalis, guaiacum, prickly ash

The following companies create formulas for cellular wellness.

### Flor-Essence

https://www.florahealth.com/

**Essiac Tea-** burdock, rumex, sheep sorrel, slippery elm, turkey rhubarb

### Shawnee Moon

https://shawneemoon.com/

**Victoria Fortner** was a master herbalist who started Shawnee Moon. After her passing, **Kerry Brock** has kept her legacy alive and continues to make these formulas based on native American and other Western herbal inspirations.

**Maskekiwapwe**- sheep sorrel aerial, burdock root, slippery elm bark, & turkey rhubarb root. (a version of the Essiac Formula)

**Immuno Boost**- suma root, peony root, gotu kola, chrysanthemum flower, astragalus root, licorice root, kelp, pau d'arco bark, red clover.

**TOF (The Other Formula)**- cat's claw bark, chaparral leaf, pau d'arco bark, astragalus root, fo-ti root, buckthorn bark, burdock root, dandelion root, echinacea root, lomatium root, osha root, parsley leaf, red clover flower, yellow dock root.

**MITOF** (all 3 of the above formulas together)- sheep sorrel, burdock root, slippery elm bark, turkey rhubarb root, pau d'arco bark, red clover flower, suma root, peony root, gotu kola aerial, chrysanthemum flower, astragalus root, licorice root, kelp, cat's claw bark, chaparral leaf, astragalus root, fo-ti root, buckthorn bark, burdock root, dandelion root, echinacea root, lomatium root, osha root, parsley leaf, yellow dock root.

## Natura Health Products

https://www.naturahealthproducts.com

Master herbalist and cancer specialist **Donnie Yance** has created many supportive plant-based formulas that include:

Botanical Treasures, Mushroom Synergy, Vital Adapt, Cell Guardian, Artemis Plus

**Econugenics**

https://econugenics.com

**Dr Issac Eliaz** has formulated a long line of supplements for detoxification and cancer support including:

Pectasol, Pectaclear, Glypho Cleanse, Ecoprobiotic, Mycophyto, Ecodetox, CellularShield, Breast Defend, ProstaCaid, Honopure

# Chapter 8 Action Steps

Write in your journal or notebook:

- Which herbs have you already heard of, or have seen at a health-food store?

- Which herbs have you never heard of that seem interesting for your situation?

- Which Herbal Formulas would you like to order or learn more about?

# Chapter 9

## The Molecular Pathway: Part 3- Supplements

*"Nutrient combinations augment each other to achieve greater healing capacity."*

-Patrick Quillin, Author of *Beating Cancer with Nutrition*

-A-

**Akkermansia muciniphila-** is a probiotic that helps you respond to cancer immunotherapy more effectively. Pomegranate and cranberry juice help you replenish this helpful bacteria. It is now also available as a supplement. The more of this probiotic that people generally have, the lower the incidence of obesity and diabetes that they have.

Cani PD, Depommier C, Derrien M, Everard A, de Vos WM. Akkermansia muciniphila: paradigm for next-generation beneficial microorganisms. Nat Rev Gastroenterol Hepatol. 2022 Oct;19(10):625-637. doi: 10.1038/s41575-022-00631-9. Epub 2022 May 31. Erratum in: Nat Rev Gastroenterol Hepatol. 2022 Jun 23;: PMID: 35641786.

Derosa L, Routy B, Thomas AM, Iebba V, Zalcman G, Friard S, Mazieres J, Audigier-Valette C, Moro-Sibilot D, Goldwasser F, Silva CAC, Terrisse S, Bonvalet M, Scherpereel A, Pegliasco H, Richard C, Ghiringhelli F, Elkrief A, Desilets A, Blanc-Durand F, Cumbo F, Blanco A, Boidot R, Chevrier S, Daillère R, Kroemer G, Alla L, Pons N, Le Chatelier E, Galleron N, Roume H, Dubuisson A, Bouchard N, Messaoudene M, Drubay D, Deutsch E, Barlesi F, Planchard D, Segata N, Martinez S, Zitvogel L, Soria JC, Besse B. Intestinal Akkermansia muciniphila predicts clinical response to PD-1 blockade in patients with advanced non-small-cell lung cancer. Nat Med. 2022 Feb;28(2):315-324. doi: 10.1038/s41591-021-01655-5. Epub 2022 Feb 3. PMID: 35115705; PMCID: PMC9330544.

Zhang T, Li Q, Cheng L, Buch H, Zhang F. Akkermansia muciniphila is a promising probiotic. Microb Biotechnol. 2019 Nov;12(6):1109-1125. doi: 10.1111/1751-7915.13410. Epub 2019 Apr 21. PMID: 31006995; PMCID: PMC6801136.

**Alpha-Lipoic Acid-** Is an antioxidant that lowers blood sugar and supports mitochondrial health. It is one of the supplements most studied for its ability to treat nerve pain induced by chemotherapy.

Dinicola S, Fuso A, Cucina A, Santiago-Reyes M, Verna R, Unfer V, Monastra G, Bizzarri M. Natural products - alpha-lipoic acid and acetyl-L-carnitine - in the treatment of chemotherapy-induced peripheral neuropathy. Eur Rev Med Pharmacol Sci. 2018 Jul;22(14):4739-4754. doi: 10.26355/eurrev_201807_15534. PMID: 30058711.

Schloss JM, Colosimo M, Airey C, Masci PP, Linnane AW, Vitetta L. Nutraceuticals and chemotherapy induced peripheral neuropathy (CIPN): a systematic review. Clin Nutr. 2013 Dec;32(6):888-93. doi: 10.1016/j.clnu.2013.04.007. Epub 2013 Apr 13. Erratum in: Clin Nutr. 2015 Feb;34(1):167. PMID: 23647723.

**Ammonium Tetrathiomolybdate (TBM)**- If you have elevated levels of copper upon testing, this molecule can bind copper and remove it from the body. Since copper is required for the creation of new blood vessels, this will help reduce the amount of angiogenesis and starve the tumor of its blood supply. In one study, TBM was shown to enhance the antitumor effect of the chemotherapy drug cisplatin in head and neck cancer.

Denoyer D, Clatworthy SAS, Cater MA. Copper Complexes in Cancer Therapy. Met Ions Life Sci. 2018 Feb 5;18:/books/9783110470734/9783110470734-022/9783110470734-022.xml. doi: 10.1515/9783110470734-022. PMID: 29394035.

Ryumon S, Okui T, Kunisada Y, Kishimoto K, Shimo T, Hasegawa K, Ibaragi S, Akiyama K, Thu Ha NT, Monsur Hassan NM, Sasaki A. Ammonium tetrathiomolybdate enhances the antitumor effect of cisplatin via the suppression of ATPase copper transporting beta in head and neck squamous cell carcinoma. Oncol Rep. 2019 Dec;42(6):2611-2621. doi: 10.3892/or.2019.7367. Epub 2019 Oct 10. PMID: 31638244; PMCID: PMC6826331.

**Apigenin**- is a natural flavonoid molecule found in certain plants, such as parsley, chamomile, and celery. Studies have shown that apigenin has anticancer properties, and may help prevent the growth and spread of cancer cells by inducing cell cycle arrest, inhibiting angiogenesis, and promoting apoptosis. Apigenin may also enhance the effectiveness of conventional cancer therapies, such as chemotherapy and radiation, while reducing their toxic side effects.

Jiang ZB, Wang WJ, Xu C, Xie YJ, Wang XR, Zhang YZ, Huang JM, Huang M, Xie C, Liu P, Fan XX, Ma YP, Yan PY, Liu L, Yao XJ, Wu QB, Lai-Han Leung E. Luteolin and its derivative apigenin suppress the inducible PD-L1 expression to improve anti-tumor immunity in KRAS-mutant lung cancer. Cancer Lett. 2021 Sep 1;515:36-48. doi: 10.1016/j.canlet.2021.05.019. Epub 2021 May 28. PMID: 34052328.

Singh D, Gupta M, Sarwat M, Siddique HR. Apigenin in cancer prevention and therapy: A systematic review and meta-analysis of animal models. Crit Rev Oncol Hematol. 2022 Aug;176:103751. doi: 10.1016/j.critrevonc.2022.103751. Epub 2022 Jun 22. PMID: 35752426.

Rahmani AH, Alsahli MA, Almatroudi A, Almogbel MA, Khan AA, Anwar S, Almatroodi SA. The Potential Role of Apigenin in Cancer Prevention and Treatment. Molecules. 2022 Sep 16;27(18):6051. doi: 10.3390/molecules27186051. PMID: 36144783; PMCID: PMC9505045.

**Artemisinin-** is a natural compound derived from the sweet wormwood plant that has been used for centuries in traditional Chinese medicine to treat fevers and malaria. In recent years, it has gained attention for its potential anti-cancer properties. Several studies and some clinical trials have suggested that artemisinin can be effective in killing cancer cells and inhibiting the growth and spread of tumors. It is thought that artemisinin may work by inducing programmed cell suicide, inducing ferroptosis (iron-dependant) cell death, and disrupting the cell growth cycle.

Chen GQ, Benthani FA, Wu J, Liang D, Bian ZX, Jiang X. Artemisinin compounds sensitize cancer cells to ferroptosis by regulating iron homeostasis. Cell Death Differ. 2020 Jan;27(1):242-254. doi: 10.1038/s41418-019-0352-3. Epub 2019 May 21. PMID: 31114026; PMCID: PMC7205875.

Kiani BH, Kayani WK, Khayam AU, Dilshad E, Ismail H, Mirza B. Artemisinin and its derivatives: a promising cancer therapy. Mol Biol Rep. 2020 Aug;47(8):6321-6336. doi: 10.1007/s11033-020-05669-z. Epub 2020 Jul 24. PMID: 32710388.

Efferth T. From ancient herb to modern drug: Artemisia annua and artemisinin for cancer therapy. Semin Cancer Biol. 2017 Oct;46:65-83. doi: 10.1016/j.semcancer.2017.02.009. Epub 2017 Feb 28. PMID: 28254675.

Hu Y, Guo N, Yang T, Yan J, Wang W, Li X. The Potential Mechanisms by which Artemisinin and Its Derivatives Induce Ferroptosis in the Treatment of Cancer. Oxid Med Cell Longev. 2022 Jan 4;2022:1458143. doi: 10.1155/2022/1458143. PMID: 35028002; PMCID: PMC8752222.

-B-

**Baicalein-** is a flavonoid compound found in Chinese Skullcap (Scutellaria baicalensis). It has been studied for its anticancer properties and has been shown to induce apoptosis and inhibit angiogenesis in cancer cells. Baicalein may also enhance the efficacy of chemotherapy drugs while reducing their toxicity.

Yu M, Qi B, Xiaoxiang W, Xu J, Liu X. Baicalein increases cisplatin sensitivity of A549 lung adenocarcinoma cells via PI3K/Akt/NF-κB pathway. Biomed Pharmacother. 2017 Jun;90:677-685. doi: 10.1016/j.biopha.2017.04.001. Epub 2017 Apr 14. PMID: 28415048.

Tuli HS, Aggarwal V, Kaur J, Aggarwal D, Parashar G, Parashar NC, Tuorkey M, Kaur G, Savla R, Sak K, Kumar M. Baicalein: A metabolite with promising antineoplastic activity. Life Sci. 2020 Oct 15;259:118183. doi: 10.1016/j.lfs.2020.118183. Epub 2020 Aug 8. PMID: 32781058.

**Bee Pollen**- contains caffeic acid and many vitamins and minerals. It also contains yet unidentified molecules that can inhibit the growth of certain cancers.

Kocot J, Kiełczykowska M, Luchowska-Kocot D, Kurzepa J, Musik I. Antioxidant Potential of Propolis, Bee Pollen, and Royal Jelly: Possible Medical Application. Oxid Med Cell Longev. 2018 May 2;2018:7074209. doi: 10.1155/2018/7074209. PMID: 29854089; PMCID: PMC5954854.

Algethami JS, El-Wahed AAA, Elashal MH, Ahmed HR, Elshafiey EH, Omar EM, Naggar YA, Algethami AF, Shou Q, Alsharif SM, Xu B, Shehata AA, Guo Z, Khalifa SAM, Wang K, El-Seedi HR. Bee Pollen: Clinical Trials and Patent Applications. Nutrients. 2022 Jul 12;14(14):2858. doi: 10.3390/nu14142858. PMID: 35889814; PMCID: PMC9323277.

**Berberine**- is a natural compound found in certain plants such as Barberry, Oregon Grape, Goldenseal, and Coptis. Studies have shown that berberine has anticancer properties and may inhibit the growth and spread of cancer cells by inducing cell cycle arrest, promoting apoptosis, and inhibiting angiogenesis. It is also used to help with blood sugar regulation and gut dysbiosis. Berberine may also enhance the effectiveness of conventional cancer therapies, such as chemotherapy and radiation, while reducing their toxic side effects.

Ortiz LM, Lombardi P, Tillhon M, Scovassi AI. Berberine, an epiphany against cancer. Molecules. 2014 Aug 15;19(8):12349-67. doi: 10.3390/molecules190812349. PMID: 25153862; PMCID: PMC6271598.

Liu L, Fan J, Ai G, Liu J, Luo N, Li C, Cheng Z. Berberine in combination with cisplatin induces necroptosis and apoptosis in ovarian cancer cells. Biol Res. 2019 Jul 18;52(1):37. doi: 10.1186/s40659-019-0243-6. PMID: 31319879; PMCID: PMC6637630.

Liu Q, Tang J, Chen S, Hu S, Shen C, Xiang J, Chen N, Wang J, Ma X, Zhang Y, Zeng J. Berberine for gastric cancer prevention and treatment: Multi-step actions on the Correa's cascade underlie its therapeutic effects. Pharmacol Res. 2022 Oct;184:106440. doi: 10.1016/j.phrs.2022.106440. Epub 2022 Sep 13. PMID: 36108874.

**Beta 1,3 Glucans**- are natural compounds found in certain plants and fungi, such as mushrooms, yeast, and oats. Studies have shown that beta 1,3 glucans have anticancer properties and can stimulate the immune system to fight cancer cells better. Beta 1,3 glucans may also enhance the effectiveness of chemotherapy and radiation therapies while reducing their side effects.

Sylla B, Legentil L, Saraswat-Ohri S, Vashishta A, Daniellou R, Wang HW, Vetvicka V, Ferrières V. Oligo-β-(1 → 3)-glucans: impact of thio-bridges on immunostimulating activities and the development of cancer stem cells. J Med Chem. 2014 Oct 23;57(20):8280-92. doi: 10.1021/jm500506b. Epub 2014 Oct 10. PMID: 25268857.

Caseiro C, Dias JNR, de Andrade Fontes CMG, Bule P. From Cancer Therapy to Winemaking: The Molecular Structure and Applications of β-Glucans and β-1, 3-Glucanases. Int J Mol Sci. 2022 Mar 15;23(6):3156. doi: 10.3390/ijms23063156. PMID: 35328577; PMCID: PMC8949617.

**Beta-sitosterol-** is a sterol molecule found in certain plants such as Saw Palmetto, Soybeans, and Pumpkin Seeds. Studies have shown that beta-sitosterol has anticancer properties and may inhibit the growth and spread of cancer cells. Beta-sitosterol may also reduce inflammation and enhance the immune system, making it a useful treatment for cancer.

Khan Z, Nath N, Rauf A, Emran TB, Mitra S, Islam F, Chandran D, Barua J, Khandaker MU, Idris AM, Wilairatana P, Thiruvengadam M. Multifunctional roles and pharmacological potential of β-sitosterol: Emerging evidence toward clinical applications. Chem Biol Interact. 2022 Sep 25;365:110117. doi: 10.1016/j.cbi.2022.110117. Epub 2022 Aug 19. PMID: 35995256.

Bin Sayeed MS, Ameen SS. Beta-Sitosterol: A Promising but Orphan Nutraceutical to Fight Against Cancer. Nutr Cancer. 2015;67(8):1214-20. doi: 10.1080/01635581.2015.1087042. Epub 2015 Oct 16. PMID: 26473555.

Bae H, Park S, Ham J, Song J, Hong T, Choi JH, Song G, Lim W. ER-Mitochondria Calcium Flux by β-Sitosterol Promotes Cell Death in Ovarian Cancer. Antioxidants (Basel). 2021 Oct 8;10(10):1583. doi: 10.3390/antiox10101583. PMID: 34679718; PMCID: PMC8533280.

**Branched Chain Amino Acids (BCAAs)-** are the essential amino acids leucine, isoleucine, and valine found in supplements and certain foods, such as meat, dairy, and legumes. Studies have shown that BCAAs help reduce cachexia or muscle wasting in cancer patients, or those undergoing chemotherapy, radiation, or surgery. BCAAs also improve immune function and reduce inflammation, making them a useful supplement for cancer patients.

Sivanand S, Vander Heiden MG. Emerging Roles for Branched-Chain Amino Acid Metabolism in Cancer. Cancer Cell. 2020 Feb 10;37(2):147-156. doi: 10.1016/j.ccell.2019.12.011. PMID: 32049045; PMCID: PMC7082774.

Neinast M, Murashige D, Arany Z. Branched Chain Amino Acids. Annu Rev Physiol. 2019 Feb 10;81:139-164. doi: 10.1146/annurev-physiol-020518-114455. Epub 2018 Nov 28. PMID: 30485760; PMCID: PMC6536377.

Ananieva EA, Wilkinson AC. Branched-chain amino acid metabolism in cancer. Curr Opin Clin Nutr Metab Care. 2018 Jan;21(1):64-70. doi: 10.1097/MCO.0000000000000430. PMID: 29211698; PMCID: PMC5732628.

**Bromelain**- is a natural enzyme found most abundantly in pineapple stems. Studies have shown that bromelain has anticancer properties and may induce apoptosis, inhibit angiogenesis, and enhance the immune system's ability to fight cancer cells. Bromelain may also enhance the effectiveness of chemotherapy and radiation therapies while reducing their side effects. It has been shown to block the inflammatory PGE2 molecule, and it can help reduce scar tissue, thrombosis, cell adhesion, and migration.

Chobotova K, Vernallis AB, Majid FA. Bromelain's activity and potential as an anti-cancer agent: Current evidence and perspectives. Cancer Lett. 2010 Apr 28;290(2):148-56. doi: 10.1016/j.canlet.2009.08.001. Epub 2009 Aug 22. PMID: 19700238.

Mekkawy AH, Pillai K, Suh H, Badar S, Akhter J, Képénékian V, Ke K, Valle SJ, Morris DL. Bromelain and acetylcysteine (BromAc®) alone and in combination with gemcitabine inhibit subcutaneous deposits of pancreatic cancer after intraperitoneal injection. Am J Transl Res. 2021 Dec 15;13(12):13524-13539. PMID: 35035694; PMCID: PMC8748110.

de Lencastre Novaes LC, Jozala AF, Lopes AM, de Carvalho Santos-Ebinuma V, Mazzola PG, Pessoa Junior A. Stability, purification, and applications of bromelain: A review. Biotechnol Prog. 2016 Jan-Feb;32(1):5-13. doi: 10.1002/btpr.2190. Epub 2015 Nov 17. PMID: 26518672.

-C-

**Calcium-D-Glucarate (CDG)**- is a natural substance found in some fruits and vegetables that has been studied for its potential role in cancer prevention and treatment. CDG has been shown to help the body eliminate toxins and excess hormones that can contribute to the development of cancer. It has also been found to inhibit the activity of an enzyme called beta-glucuronidase, which can promote the growth and spread of cancer cells. Studies have suggested that CDG may be particularly effective in preventing hormone-related cancers, such as breast and prostate cancer. In addition, CDG has been found to enhance the effectiveness of chemotherapy drugs and reduce their side effects.

Heerdt AS, Young CW, Borgen PI. Calcium glucarate as a chemopreventive agent in breast cancer. Isr J Med Sci. 1995 Feb-Mar;31(2-3):101-5. PMID: 7744577.

Walaszek Z, Szemraj J, Narog M, Adams AK, Kilgore J, Sherman U, Hanausek M. Metabolism, uptake, and excretion of a D-glucaric acid salt and its potential use in cancer prevention. Cancer Detect Prev. 1997;21(2):178-90. PMID: 9101079.

**Cartilage-** Cartilage supplements have been used for several decades as an alternative cancer treatment. The concept is that cartilage contains anti-angiogenesis molecules that prevent cancer tumors from forming new blood vessels and thus starving them of nutrients. Shark cartilage was extensively used and recommended in the 80's and 90's but due to price and environmental concerns and lack of scientific documentation it has generally fallen out of favor, and more affordable bovine (cow) and other forms of cartilage seem to have more evidence for antiangiogenic effects.

Wu R, Li P, Wang Y, Su N, Xiao M, Li X, Shang N. Structural analysis and anti-cancer activity of low-molecular-weight chondroitin sulfate from hybrid sturgeon cartilage. Carbohydr Polym. 2022 Jan 1;275:118700. doi: 10.1016/j.carbpol.2021.118700. Epub 2021 Sep 24. PMID: 34742426.

Patra D, Sandell LJ. Antiangiogenic and anticancer molecules in cartilage. Expert Rev Mol Med. 2012 Jan 19;14:e10. doi: 10.1017/erm.2012.3. PMID: 22559283.

Prudden JF. The treatment of human cancer with agents prepared from bovine cartilage. J Biol Response Mod. 1985 Dec;4(6):551-84. PMID: 4087031.

**Coenzyme Q-10-** is a naturally occurring antioxidant synthesized by the liver that plays a critical role in the production of energy within cells. It has been studied for its potential role in cancer prevention and treatment due to its ability to protect cells from damage caused by free radicals and support immune function. CoQ10 has been found to inhibit the growth and spread of cancer cells in laboratory studies and animal models. Several clinical studies have also suggested that CoQ10 supplementation may improve outcomes in cancer patients, particularly those undergoing chemotherapy or radiation therapy. It has been found to reduce the severity of side effects such as fatigue and nausea, and may also enhance the effectiveness of these treatments.

Arenas-Jal M, Suñé-Negre JM, García-Montoya E. Coenzyme Q10 supplementation: Efficacy, safety, and formulation challenges. Compr Rev Food Sci Food Saf. 2020 Mar;19(2):574-594. doi: 10.1111/1541-4337.12539. Epub 2020 Feb 19. PMID: 33325173.

Koppula P, Lei G, Zhang Y, Yan Y, Mao C, Kondiparthi L, Shi J, Liu X, Horbath A, Das M, Li W, Poyurovsky MV, Olszewski K, Gan B. A targetable CoQ-FSP1 axis drives ferroptosis- and radiation-resistance in KEAP1 inactive lung cancers. Nat Commun. 2022 Apr 22;13(1):2206. doi: 10.1038/s41467-022-29905-1. PMID: 35459868; PMCID: PMC9033817.

**Chrysin-** is a flavonoid found in nature such as in passionflower, chrysanthemum, calendula, honey, and propolis. It has been studied for its potential anti-cancer properties due to its ability to inhibit the growth and spread of cancer cells in laboratory studies and animal models. Chrysin has been found to induce cell death in cancer cells and inhibit the activity of enzymes that promote cancer growth. Studies have suggested that chrysin may be particularly effective in preventing and treating hormone-related cancers, such as breast and prostate cancer, by blocking the action of estrogen.

Kasala ER, Bodduluru LN, Madana RM, V AK, Gogoi R, Barua CC. Chemopreventive and therapeutic potential of chrysin in cancer: mechanistic perspectives. Toxicol Lett. 2015 Mar 4;233(2):214-25. doi: 10.1016/j.toxlet.2015.01.008. Epub 2015 Jan 14. PMID: 25596314.

Salama AAA, Allam RM. Promising targets of chrysin and daidzein in colorectal cancer: Amphiregulin, CXCL1, and MMP-9. Eur J Pharmacol. 2021 Feb 5;892:173763. doi: 10.1016/j.ejphar.2020.173763. Epub 2020 Nov 27. PMID: 33249075.

**Chlorella**- is a type of single-celled green algae that is often used as a dietary supplement due to its high nutrient content. It has been studied for its potential anti-cancer properties, as it contains compounds such as chlorophyll and carotenoids that have antioxidant and anti-inflammatory effects. Some laboratory studies have suggested that chlorella may inhibit the growth of cancer cells and induce cell death. In animal studies, chlorella has been found to enhance the immune system's response to cancer cells and reduce the incidence and growth of tumors. It may also naturally increase albumin levels, which is associated with better outcomes in cancer.

Lemieszek MK, Rzeski W. Enhancement of chemopreventive properties of young green barley and chlorella extracts used together against colon cancer cells. Ann Agric Environ Med. 2020 Dec 22;27(4):591-598. doi: 10.26444/aaem/130555. Epub 2020 Nov 30. PMID: 33356066.

Zhang J, Liu L, Chen F. Production and characterization of exopolysaccharides from Chlorella zofingiensis and Chlorella vulgaris with anti-colorectal cancer activity. Int J Biol Macromol. 2019 Aug 1;134:976-983. doi: 10.1016/j.ijbiomac.2019.05.117. Epub 2019 May 21. PMID: 31121230.

-D-

**Delphinidin**- is a type of flavonoid in the anthocyanin family, a group of naturally occurring pigments found in many fruits and vegetables. It has been studied for its potential anti-cancer properties due to its ability to inhibit the growth and spread of cancer cells in laboratory studies and animal models. Delphinidin has been found to induce cell death in cancer cells and inhibit the activity of enzymes that promote cancer growth. It may be particularly effective in preventing and treating certain types of cancer, such as colon and breast cancer. It has been found to have antioxidant and anti-inflammatory effects that may protect cells from damage and reduce the risk of cancer.

Sharma A, Choi HK, Kim YK, Lee HJ. Delphinidin and Its Glycosides' War on Cancer: Preclinical Perspectives. Int J Mol Sci. 2021 Oct 25;22(21):11500. doi: 10.3390/ijms222111500. PMID: 34768930; PMCID: PMC8583959.

Peng J, Wu A, Yu X, Zhong Q, Deng X, Zhu Y. Combined Network Pharmacology and Cytology Experiments to Identify Potential Anti-Breast Cancer Targets and Mechanisms of Delphinidin. Nutr Cancer. 2022;74(7):2591-2606. doi: 10.1080/01635581.2021.2012582. Epub 2021 Dec 8. PMID: 34875956.

**Docosahexaenoic acid (DHA)**- is an omega-3 fatty acid found in fatty fish and algae and is one of the foundational nutrient molecules for almost all life on earth. It has been studied for its potential role in cancer prevention and treatment due to its anti-inflammatory and anti-proliferative properties. DHA has been found to inhibit the growth and spread of cancer cells in laboratory studies and animal models. Some clinical studies have suggested that DHA supplementation may improve outcomes in cancer patients, particularly those with breast, colon, and prostate cancer. It has been found to reduce inflammation, enhance immune function, and enhance the effectiveness of chemotherapy and radiation therapy.

Song EA, Kim H. Docosahexaenoic Acid Induces Oxidative DNA Damage and Apoptosis, and Enhances the Chemosensitivity of Cancer Cells. Int J Mol Sci. 2016 Aug 3;17(8):1257. doi: 10.3390/ijms17081257. PMID: 27527148; PMCID: PMC5000655.

Zhao H, Wu S, Luo Z, Liu H, Sun J, Jin X. The association between circulating docosahexaenoic acid and lung cancer: A Mendelian randomization study. Clin Nutr. 2022 Nov;41(11):2529-2536. doi: 10.1016/j.clnu.2022.09.004. Epub 2022 Sep 16. PMID: 36223714.

Fabian CJ, Kimler BF, Hursting SD. Omega-3 fatty acids for breast cancer prevention and survivorship. Breast Cancer Res. 2015 May 4;17(1):62. doi: 10.1186/s13058-015-0571-6. PMID: 25936773; PMCID: PMC4418048.

Kuban-Jankowska A, Gorska-Ponikowska M, Sahu KK, Kostrzewa T, Wozniak M, Tuszynski J. Docosahexaenoic Acid Inhibits PTP1B Phosphatase and the Viability of MCF-7 Breast Cancer Cells. Nutrients. 2019 Oct 23;11(11):2554. doi: 10.3390/nu11112554. PMID: 31652764; PMCID: PMC6893741.

**DHEA Cream**- According to Dr Jonathan Wright, DHEA has the power to downregulate a key enzyme that cancer cells use to make energy. This enzyme is called glucose-6-phosphate dehydrogenase (G6PD). It is important to use topical cream instead of DHEA pills because the liver transforms this hormone when it is taken through the stomach into other undesirable forms of the hormone.

Somers, Suzanne. *Knockout.* Crown Archetype, 2009.

**Diindolylmethane (DIM)**- is a compound that is formed when the body breaks down indole-3-carbinol, a substance found in cruciferous vegetables such as broccoli and cauliflower. DIM has been studied for its potential anti-cancer properties, as it has been found to inhibit the growth and spread of cancer cells in laboratory studies and animal models. It has anti-inflammatory and anti-angiogenic effects, which may contribute to its anti-cancer activity. It has also been found to enhance the immune system's response to cancer cells and increase the effectiveness of chemo and radiation therapy.

R, Bargil S, Ber Y, Ozlavo R, Sivan T, Rapson Y, Pomerantz A, Tsoref D, Sharon E, Caspi O, Grubsrein A, Margel D. 3,3-Diindolylmethane (DIM): a nutritional intervention and its impact on breast density in healthy BRCA carriers. A prospective clinical trial. Carcinogenesis. 2020 Oct 15;41(10):1395-1401. doi: 10.1093/carcin/bgaa050. PMID: 32458980; PMCID: PMC7566319.

Thomson CA, Ho E, Strom MB. Chemopreventive properties of 3,3'-diindolylmethane in breast cancer: evidence from experimental and human studies. Nutr Rev. 2016 Jul;74(7):432-43. doi: 10.1093/nutrit/nuw010. Epub 2016 May 31. PMID: 27261275; PMCID: PMC5059820.

**Deuterium Depleted Water (DDW)**- Deuterium is a naturally-occurring heavier isotope of hydrogen that can be found in water and other compounds. Deuterium-depleted water is water that has a lower concentration of deuterium than normal water. DDW has been studied for its potential role in cancer treatment and prevention, as higher levels of deuterium have been linked to cancer growth. Studies have shown that DDW can inhibit the growth and spread of cancer cells, and may enhance the effectiveness of chemotherapy and radiation. Some clinical studies have also suggested that DDW may improve outcomes in cancer patients.

See https://www.ddcenters.com for more information.

Wang H, Zhu B, He Z, Fu H, Dai Z, Huang G, Li B, Qin D, Zhang X, Tian L, Fang W, Yang H. Deuterium-depleted water (DDW) inhibits the proliferation and migration of nasopharyngeal carcinoma cells in vitro. Biomed Pharmacother. 2013 Jul;67(6):489-96. doi: 10.1016/j.biopha.2013.02.001. Epub 2013 Feb 27. PMID: 23773852.

Gyöngyi Z, Budán F, Szabó I, Ember I, Kiss I, Krempels K, Somlyai I, Somlyai G. Deuterium depleted water effects on survival of lung cancer patients and expression of Kras, Bcl2, and Myc genes in mouse lung. Nutr Cancer. 2013;65(2):240-6. doi: 10.1080/01635581.2013.756533. PMID: 23441611; PMCID: PMC3613976.

Yavari K, Kooshesh L. Deuterium Depleted Water Inhibits the Proliferation of Human MCF7 Breast Cancer Cell Lines by Inducing Cell Cycle Arrest. Nutr Cancer. 2019;71(6):1019-1029. doi: 10.1080/01635581.2019.1595048. Epub 2019 May 2. PMID: 31045450.

Wang H, Liu C, Fang W, Yang H. [Research progress of the inhibitory effect of deuterium-depleted water on cancers]. Nan Fang Yi Ke Da Xue Xue Bao. 2012 Oct;32(10):1454-6. Chinese. PMID: 23076183.

-E-

**Ellagic Acid**- is a natural polyphenol compound found in various fruits, nuts, and vegetables, such as raspberries, strawberries, pomegranates, and walnuts. It has been studied for its anti-cancer properties, as it has been found to inhibit the growth and spread of cancer cells in lab studies. Ellagic acid has been shown to have antioxidant and anti-inflammatory effects, which may contribute to its anti-cancer activity. It has also been found to enhance the immune system's response to cancer cells and increase the effectiveness of chemo and radiation therapy.

Xue P, Zhang G, Zhang J, Ren L. Synergism of ellagic acid in combination with radiotherapy and chemotherapy for cancer treatment. Phytomedicine. 2022 Feb 18;99:153998. doi: 10.1016/j.phymed.2022.153998. Epub ahead of print. PMID: 35217437.

Ceci C, Lacal PM, Tentori L, De Martino MG, Miano R, Graziani G. Experimental Evidence of the Antitumor, Antimetastatic and Antiangiogenic Activity of Ellagic Acid. Nutrients. 2018 Nov 14;10(11):1756. doi: 10.3390/nu10111756. PMID: 30441769; PMCID: PMC6266224.

Ceci C, Tentori L, Atzori MG, Lacal PM, Bonanno E, Scimeca M, Cicconi R, Mattei M, de Martino MG, Vespasiani G, Miano R, Graziani G. Ellagic Acid Inhibits Bladder Cancer Invasiveness and In Vivo Tumor Growth. Nutrients. 2016 Nov 22;8(11):744. doi: 10.3390/nu8110744. PMID: 27879653; PMCID: PMC5133127.

**Estriol**- also known as E3, is the most cancer-protective form of estrogen. Work with your doctor to evaluate your ratios of estrone, estradiol, and estriol to make sure that you have a healthy level of estriol for its anti-cancer benefits. Topical cream can be prescribed through a compounding pharmacy with your personalized ratios for hormone replacement or cancer protection.

Sánchez-Rovira P, Hirschberg AL, Gil-Gil M, Bermejo-De Las Heras B, Nieto-Magro C. A Phase II Prospective, Randomized, Double-Blind, Placebo-Controlled and Multicenter Clinical Trial to Assess the Safety of 0.005% Estriol Vaginal Gel in Hormone Receptor-Positive Postmenopausal Women with Early Stage Breast Cancer in Treatment with Aromatase Inhibitor in the Adjuvant Setting. Oncologist. 2020 Dec;25(12):e1846-1854. doi: 10.1634/theoncologist.2020-0417. Epub 2020 Jun 9. PMID: 32459035; PMCID: PMC8108054.

Buchholz S, Mögele M, Lintermans A, Bellen G, Prasauskas V, Ortmann O, Grob P, Neven P, Donders G. Vaginal estriol-lactobacilli combination and quality of life in endocrine-treated breast cancer. Climacteric. 2015 Apr;18(2):252-9. doi: 10.3109/13697137.2014.991301. Epub 2015 Jan 20. PMID: 25427450.

Katzenellenbogen BS. Biology and receptor interactions of estriol and estriol derivatives in vitro and in vivo. J Steroid Biochem. 1984 Apr;20(4B):1033-7. doi: 10.1016/0022-4731(84)90015-3. PMID: 6727348.

**Estrogen Ratios**- While this is not a supplement, it is a critical concept to understand, especially for breast and prostate cancers. In functional hormone urine testing such as the DUTCH Test, ratios are measured for different forms of estrogen that have either cancer protective or cancer promoting effects. The 2 forms of estrogen that are protective are easy to remember because they both start with 2: (Just remember, with estrogen, "2 is all you want to do") These are 2-hydroxy estrogen and 2-methoxy estrogen. You can help nourish the pathway to make more 2-hydroxy estrogen by eating more foods from the Brassica family (Broccoli, Cauliflower, Kale, Cabbage, Bok Choy, etc). The supplements Indole-3-carbinol (I3C) and Diindolylmethane (DIM) are concentrated sources that also promote the 2-hydroxy estrogen pathway. You can stimulate the production of more of the protective 2-methoxy estrogen by eating more green leafy vegetables, nuts, seeds, and beets. Supplements such as methyl folate (active vitamin B-9) methylcobalamin (active B-12), and Trimethylglycine (TMG), can also promote the healthy 2-methoxy estrogen pathway.

Ziegler RG, Fuhrman BJ, Moore SC, Matthews CE. Epidemiologic studies of estrogen metabolism and breast cancer. Steroids. 2015 Jul;99(Pt A):67-75. doi: 10.1016/j.steroids.2015.02.015. Epub 2015 Feb 26. PMID: 25725255; PMCID: PMC5722219.

-F-

**Fenbendazole**- is a broad-spectrum antiparasitic drug that is commonly used in veterinary medicine to treat intestinal parasites in animals. However, in recent years, it has gained attention for its potential anti-cancer properties. Some laboratory studies and case reports have suggested that fenbendazole may inhibit the growth and spread of cancer cells, particularly in certain types of cancer such as melanoma and lung cancer. It is thought that fenbendazole may work by inhibiting the energy production of cancer cells and inducing cell death. You can find many videos on Youtube.com under "Joe Tippens Cancer Protocol", and Fenbendazole is currently available on Amazon.com without a prescription.

Dogra N, Kumar A, Mukhopadhyay T. Fenbendazole acts as a moderate microtubule destabilizing agent and causes cancer cell death by modulating multiple cellular pathways. Sci Rep. 2018 Aug 9;8(1):11926. doi: 10.1038/s41598-018-30158-6. PMID: 30093705; PMCID: PMC6085345.

Park D, Lee JH, Yoon SP. Anti-cancer effects of fenbendazole on 5-fluorouracil-resistant colorectal cancer cells. Korean J Physiol Pharmacol. 2022 Sep 1;26(5):377-387. doi: 10.4196/kjpp.2022.26.5.377. PMID: 36039738; PMCID: PMC9437363.

Son DS, Lee ES, Adunyah SE. The Antitumor Potentials of Benzimidazole Anthelmintics as Repurposing Drugs. Immune Netw. 2020 Aug 4;20(4):e29. doi: 10.4110/in.2020.20.e29. PMID: 32895616; PMCID: PMC7458798.

**Fermented Wheat Germ Extract (FWGE) (Brand Names include Avemar and Metatrol)**- is a dietary supplement that is derived from the germ of wheat kernels that have been fermented with baker's yeast. It has been studied for its potential role in cancer treatment and prevention, as it contains several bioactive compounds that have been found to have anti-cancer properties.

Laboratory studies and some clinical trials have suggested that FWGE may enhance the effectiveness of chemotherapy and radiation, and may also inhibit the growth and spread of cancer cells. It is thought that FWGE may work by activating the immune system's response to cancer cells, inducing cancer cell suicide, and reducing inflammation in the body.

Boros LG, Nichelatti M, Shoenfeld Y. Fermented wheat germ extract (Avemar) in the treatment of cancer and autoimmune diseases. Ann N Y Acad Sci. 2005 Jun;1051:529-42. doi: 10.1196/annals.1361.097. PMID: 16126993.

Weitzen R, Epstein N, Oberman B, Shevetz R, Hidvegi M, Berger R. Fermented Wheat Germ Extract (FWGE) as a Treatment Additive for Castration-Resistant Prostate Cancer: A Pilot Clinical Trial. Nutr Cancer. 2022;74(4):1338-1346. doi: 10.1080/01635581.2021.1952457. Epub 2021 Jul 21. PMID: 34286638.

Zhurakivska K, Risteli M, Salo T, Sartini D, Salvucci A, Troiano G, Lo Muzio L, Emanuelli M. Effects of Fermented Wheat Germ Extract on Oral Cancer Cells: An In Vitro Study. Nutr Cancer. 2022;74(6):2133-2141. doi: 10.1080/01635581.2021.1976806. Epub 2021 Sep 12. PMID: 34514913.

**Ferroptosis-** is a form of regulated cell death that is characterized by the accumulation of iron and lipid peroxides in cells. It has been studied for its potential role in cancer treatment and prevention, as some cancer cells are more susceptible to ferroptosis than normal cells.

Several studies have suggested that inducing ferroptosis in cancer cells may be a promising strategy for cancer therapy, as it may lead to selective death of cancer cells while sparing normal cells. One of the main natural compounds being studied and used to induce ferroptosis is **Artemisinin**. See the Artemisinin entry in the "A" section above for more information.

Mou Y, Wang J, Wu J, He D, Zhang C, Duan C, Li B. Ferroptosis, a new form of cell death: opportunities and challenges in cancer. J Hematol Oncol. 2019 Mar 29;12(1):34. doi: 10.1186/s13045-019-0720-y. PMID: 30925886; PMCID: PMC6441206.

Zhao L, Zhou X, Xie F, Zhang L, Yan H, Huang J, Zhang C, Zhou F, Chen J, Zhang L. Ferroptosis in cancer and cancer immunotherapy. Cancer Commun (Lond). 2022 Feb;42(2):88-116. doi: 10.1002/cac2.12250. PMID: 35133083; PMCID: PMC8822596.

**Flavonoids-** are plant molecules that usually have "-in" at the end, such as: curcumin, catechin, quercetin, hesperidin, and rutin. They work better when grouped together in symphonies of flavonoids. Each flavonoid tends to target specific tissues. They team up with glutathione and other antioxidants in the body. They can block the proteolytic enzymes (MMPs) that start metastasis. Delphinidin is one of most potent flavonoids studied for cancer so far. There are hundreds of different single and complex flavonoid supplements available, but the easiest way of consuming flavonoids is to eat brightly-colored rainbow foods raw, or in fresh juices, smoothies, salads, stir fries, and soups.

Kashyap D, Garg VK, Tuli HS, Yerer MB, Sak K, Sharma AK, Kumar M, Aggarwal V, Sandhu SS. Fisetin and Quercetin: Promising Flavonoids with Chemopreventive Potential. Biomolecules. 2019 May 6;9(5):174. doi: 10.3390/biom9050174. PMID: 31064104; PMCID: PMC6572624.

Li G, Ding K, Qiao Y, Zhang L, Zheng L, Pan T, Zhang L. Flavonoids Regulate Inflammation and Oxidative Stress in Cancer. Molecules. 2020 Nov 30;25(23):5628. doi: 10.3390/molecules25235628. PMID: 33265939; PMCID: PMC7729519.

Chang H, Lei L, Zhou Y, Ye F, Zhao G. Dietary Flavonoids and the Risk of Colorectal Cancer: An Updated Meta-Analysis of Epidemiological Studies. Nutrients. 2018 Jul 23;10(7):950. doi: 10.3390/nu10070950. PMID: 30041489; PMCID: PMC6073812.

Selvakumar P, Badgeley A, Murphy P, Anwar H, Sharma U, Lawrence K, Lakshmikutty Amma A. Flavonoids and Other Polyphenols Act as Epigenetic Modifiers in Breast Cancer. Nutrients. 2020 Mar 13;12(3):761. doi: 10.3390/nu12030761. PMID: 32183060; PMCID: PMC7146477.

-G-

**Gamma Linolenic Acid (GLA)**- this is an essential fatty acid found most often in borage and evening primrose oil supplements. It can act as a natural 5-alpha-reductase inhibitor. This is the enzyme that converts testosterone into the more prostate-cancer-promoting Di-hydrotestosterone (DHT).

Wang Y, Shi J, Gong L. Gamma linolenic acid suppresses hypoxia-induced gastric cancer cell growth and epithelial-mesenchymal transition by inhibiting the Wnt/b-catenin signaling pathway. Folia Histochem Cytobiol. 2020;58(2):117-126. doi: 10.5603/FHC.a2020.0012. Epub 2020 Jul 1. PMID: 32608501.

González-Fernández MJ, Ortea I, Guil-Guerrero JL. α-Linolenic and γ-linolenic acids exercise differential antitumor effects on HT-29 human colorectal cancer cells. Toxicol Res (Camb). 2020 Jul 27;9(4):474-483. doi: 10.1093/toxres/tfaa046. PMID: 32905142; PMCID: PMC7467275.

**Genistein**- This is an isoflavone molecule found in soy. Soy is almost always discouraged by oncologists for hormone receptor positive cancers, but recent research shows that this is a medical myth, and that it really helps to block estrogen's effects at the receptor level. Several laboratory studies and some clinical trials have suggested that genistein may be effective in inhibiting the growth and spread of certain types of cancer, including breast, prostate, and colon. It is thought that genistein may work by blocking the action of enzymes that promote cancer cell growth, as well as by inducing programmed cell death in cancer cells. If soy foods or supplements are consumed, be sure that they are labeled as organic and non-GMO.

Mukund V. Genistein: Its Role in Breast Cancer Growth and Metastasis. Curr Drug Metab. 2020;21(1):6-10. doi: 10.2174/1389200221666200120121919. PMID: 31987018.

Varinska L, Gal P, Mojzisova G, Mirossay L, Mojzis J. Soy and breast cancer: focus on angiogenesis. Int J Mol Sci. 2015 May 22;16(5):11728-49. doi: 10.3390/ijms160511728. PMID: 26006245; PMCID: PMC4463727.

Bhat SS, Prasad SK, Shivamallu C, Prasad KS, Syed A, Reddy P, Cull CA, Amachawadi RG. Genistein: A Potent Anti-Breast Cancer Agent. Curr Issues Mol Biol. 2021 Oct 10;43(3):1502-1517. doi: 10.3390/cimb43030106. PMID: 34698063; PMCID: PMC8929066.

Ullah MF, Ahmad A, Zubair H, Khan HY, Wang Z, Sarkar FH, Hadi SM. Soy isoflavone genistein induces cell death in breast cancer cells through mobilization of endogenous copper ions and generation of reactive oxygen species. Mol Nutr Food Res. 2011 Apr;55(4):553-9. doi: 10.1002/mnfr.201000329. Epub 2010 Dec 6. PMID: 21462322.

**Germanium**- Is a mineral that stimulates the immune system, increases the anticancer molecule interferon, stimulates the production of natural killer cells and other white blood cells. It is an efficient carrier of oxygen into the cells. It has been shown to aid the recovery of lost weight from chemo or radiation therapy, slow tumor growth, reduce metastasis, and prolong survival times. Ginseng, garlic, aloe, and medicinal mushrooms are all high in germanium.

Kaplan BJ, Parish WW, Andrus GM, Simpson JS, Field CJ. Germane facts about germanium sesquioxide: I. Chemistry and anticancer properties. J Altern Complement Med. 2004 Apr;10(2):337-44. doi: 10.1089/107555304323062329. PMID: 15165414.

Mertens RT, Parkin S, Awuah SG. Exploring six-coordinate germanium(IV)-diketonate complexes as anticancer agents. Inorganica Chim Acta. 2020 Apr;503(1):119375. doi: 10.1016/j.ica.2019.119375. Epub 2019 Dec 19. PMID: 34565828; PMCID: PMC8460083.

**Glandulars**- Dried, purified, glandular extracts from organically raised animals, can provide natural vitamins, minerals, hormones, and peptides that provide benefits for human health. Glandular support is available for the liver, kidneys, thyroid, thymus, pancreas, adrenal, pineal, and more. The liver, thyroid, thymus, and pancreas all have biochemical influences on the cancer and immune process.

Badr El-Din NK, Othman AI, Amer ME, Ghoneum M. Thymax, a gross thymic extract, exerts cell cycle arrest and apoptosis in Ehrlich ascites carcinoma in vivo. Heliyon. 2022 Mar 5;8(3):e09047. doi: 10.1016/j.heliyon.2022.e09047. PMID: 35299600; PMCID: PMC8920936.

Bartsch H, Bartsch C, Simon WE, Flehmig B, Ebels I, Lippert TH. Antitumor activity of the pineal gland: effect of unidentified substances versus the effect of melatonin. Oncology. 1992;49(1):27-30. doi: 10.1159/000227005. PMID: 1542489.

**Grape Seed Extract**- is a natural supplement that is rich in antioxidants, including oligomeric proanthocyanidins (OPCs) and resveratrol, which have been studied for their potential role in cancer prevention and treatment. Some lab and animal studies show that grape seed extract has anti-cancer properties, as it can inhibit the growth and spread of cancer cells and induce programmed cell death in cancerous cells.

Kaur M, Agarwal C, Agarwal R. Anticancer and cancer chemopreventive potential of grape seed extract and other grape-based products. J Nutr. 2009 Sep;139(9):1806S-12S. doi: 10.3945/jn.109.106864. Epub 2009 Jul 29. PMID: 19640973; PMCID: PMC2728696.

Mancini M, Cerny MEV, Cardoso NS, Verissimo G, Maluf SW. Grape Seed Components as Protectors of Inflammation, DNA Damage, and Cancer. Curr Nutr Rep. 2023 Mar;12(1):141-150. doi: 10.1007/s13668-023-00460-5. Epub 2023 Jan 24. PMID: 36692807.

Habib HM, El-Fakharany EM, Kheadr E, Ibrahim WH. Grape seed proanthocyanidin extract inhibits DNA and protein damage and labile iron, enzyme, and cancer cell activities. Sci Rep. 2022 Jul 20;12(1):12393. doi: 10.1038/s41598-022-16608-2. PMID: 35859159; PMCID: PMC9300616.

-H-

**Honokiol**- is a natural compound found in magnolia bark, which has been studied for its anti-cancer properties. Some studies have suggested that honokiol inhibits the growth and spread of cancer cells, induces apoptosis in cancer cells, and enhances the efficacy of chemo and radiation therapy.

Pan J, Lee Y, Wang Y, You M. Honokiol targets mitochondria to halt cancer progression and metastasis. Mol Nutr Food Res. 2016 Jun;60(6):1383-95. doi: 10.1002/mnfr.201501007. Epub 2016 May 6. PMID: 27276215.

Arora S, Singh S, Piazza GA, Contreras CM, Panyam J, Singh AP. Honokiol: a novel natural agent for cancer prevention and therapy. Curr Mol Med. 2012 Dec;12(10):1244-52. doi: 10.2174/156652412803833508. PMID: 22834827; PMCID: PMC3663139.

Wang J, Liu D, Guan S, Zhu W, Fan L, Zhang Q, Cai D. Hyaluronic acid-modified liposomal honokiol nanocarrier: Enhance anti-metastasis and antitumor efficacy against breast cancer. Carbohydr Polym. 2020 May 1;235:115981. doi: 10.1016/j.carbpol.2020.115981. Epub 2020 Feb 11. PMID: 32122511.

**Hydrogen Water**- A report stated that, "A randomized, placebo-controlled study showed that consumption of hydrogen-rich water reduces the biological reaction to radiation-induced oxidative stress without compromising anti-tumor effects." Hydrogen water is available in 2 main forms: either a machine that infuses hydrogen molecules into water, or as tablets you can dissolve into a water bottle with the lid on, and this diffuses the hydrogen into the water. This is an exciting supplement that has a growing body of health research behind it.

Qian L, Shen J, Chuai Y, Cai J. Hydrogen as a new class of radioprotective agent. Int J Biol Sci. 2013 Sep 14;9(9):887-94. doi: 10.7150/ijbs.7220. PMID: 24155664; PMCID: PMC3805896.

Yang Y, Liu PY, Bao W, Chen SJ, Wu FS, Zhu PY. Hydrogen inhibits endometrial cancer growth via a ROS/NLRP3/caspase-1/GSDMD-mediated pyroptotic pathway. BMC Cancer. 2020 Jan 10;20(1):28. doi: 10.1186/s12885-019-6491-6. PMID: 31924176; PMCID: PMC6954594.

Yang N, Gong F, Liu B, Hao Y, Chao Y, Lei H, Yang X, Gong Y, Wang X, Liu Z, Cheng L. Magnesium galvanic cells produce hydrogen and modulate the tumor microenvironment to inhibit cancer growth. Nat Commun. 2022 Apr 28;13(1):2336. doi: 10.1038/s41467-022-29938-6. PMID: 35484138; PMCID: PMC9051066.

-I-

**Inositol-6-phosphate (IP6)-** is a natural compound that plays an important role in cellular signaling pathways. Some lab and animal studies have suggested that inositol-6-phosphate has anti-cancer properties, as it can inhibit the growth and spread of cancer cells, induce programmed cell death in cancer cells, block angiogenesis, and enhance the efficacy of chemotherapy and radiation.

Dorsey M, Benghuzzi H, Tucci M, Cason Z. Growth and cell viability of estradiol and IP-6 treated Hep-2 laryngeal carcinoma cells. Biomed Sci Instrum. 2005;41:205-10. PMID: 15850106.

Schneider JG, Alosi JA, McDonald DE, McFadden DW. Effects of pterostilbene on melanoma alone and in synergy with inositol hexaphosphate. Am J Surg. 2009 Nov;198(5):679-84. doi: 10.1016/j.amjsurg.2009.07.014. PMID: 19887199.

**Iodine-** Helps prevent breast cancer and other cancer processes. Iodine stimulates the conversion of the more cancer-promoting estrone and estradiol to the more protective estriol form. Iodine combines with fats to create iodo-lipids that are incorporated into the breast tissue and help kill cancer cells. It is an essential nutrient and is critical for healthy thyroid function which is also protective against the cancer process. Traditional Japanese diets contain 2-4 times more iodine than average Western countries, and they have some of the lowest levels of cancer compared to these nations. Iodine is best found in seafood & sea vegetables such as kelp, bladderwrack, and dulse.

Feldt-Rasmussen U. Iodine and cancer. Thyroid. 2001 May;11(5):483-6. doi: 10.1089/105072501300176435. PMID: 11396706.

Smyth PP. The thyroid, iodine and breast cancer. Breast Cancer Res. 2003;5(5):235-8. doi: 10.1186/bcr638. Epub 2003 Jul 29. PMID: 12927031; PMCID: PMC314438.

Eskin BA. Iodine and mammary cancer. Adv Exp Med Biol. 1977;91:293-304. doi: 10.1007/978-1-4684-0796-9_20. PMID: 343535.

**iRGD-** is a cyclic peptide (small piece of protein) that enhances the effects of chemotherapy specifically to cancer cells only. It has shown potential for improving cancer drug delivery to tumor cells. It works by binding to a specific receptor on the surface of tumor blood vessels, which allows it to penetrate deep into the tumor tissue and release its cargo of drugs directly to cancer cells. Studies have shown that iRGD can enhance the effectiveness of chemotherapy and radiation in various types of cancer, including breast and pancreatic.

Zuo H. iRGD: A Promising Peptide for Cancer Imaging and a Potential Therapeutic Agent for Various Cancers. J Oncol. 2019 Jun 26;2019:9367845. doi: 10.1155/2019/9367845. PMID: 31346334; PMCID: PMC6617877.

Yin H, Yang J, Zhang Q, Yang J, Wang H, Xu J, Zheng J. iRGD as a tumor-penetrating peptide for cancer therapy (Review). Mol Med Rep. 2017 May;15(5):2925-2930. doi: 10.3892/mmr.2017.6419. Epub 2017 Mar 30. PMID: 28358432.

Amrollahi-Nia R, Akbari V, Shafiee F. DFF40-iRGD, a novel chimeric protein with efficient cytotoxic and apoptotic effects against triple-negative breast cancer cells. Biotechnol Lett. 2021 Oct;43(10):1967-1976. doi: 10.1007/s10529-021-03178-y. Epub 2021 Sep 5. PMID: 34482510.

**Isoprinosine**- is an immunomodulating agent that has been used in the treatment of various viral and immunodeficiency disorders. However, recent research has also suggested that it has potential in the treatment and prevention of certain types of cancer. Isoprinosine has been found to modulate immune function and inhibit the growth and proliferation of cancer cells in vitro and in animal models. Clinical studies have shown promising results in the treatment of several types of cancer, including cervical, breast, and leukemia. It has also been found to enhance the efficacy of chemo and radiation therapy.

Simon LN, Hoehler FK, McKenzie DT, Hadden JW. Isoprinosine and NPT 15392: immunomodulation and cancer. Adv Exp Med Biol. 1983;166:241-59. doi: 10.1007/978-1-4757-1410-4_20. PMID: 6196956.

Tobólska S, Terpiłowska S, Jaroszewski J, Siwicki AK. Influence of Inosine Pranobex on Cell Viability in Normal Fibroblasts and Liver Cancer Cells. J Vet Res. 2018 Oct 24;62(2):215-220. doi: 10.2478/jvetres-2018-0031. PMID: 30364913; PMCID: PMC6200297.

Colozza M, Tonato M, Belsanti V, Mosconi AM, Fiorucci S, Gernini I, Rambotti P, Davis S. 5-Fluorouracil and isoprinosine in the treatment of advanced colorectal cancer. A limited phase I, II evaluation. Cancer. 1988 Sep 15;62(6):1049-52. doi: 10.1002/1097-0142(19880915)62:6<1049::aid-cncr2820620604>3.0.co;2-k. PMID: 2457421.

-K-

**Ketones**- (Pruvit KETO/OS, Kegenix, etc)- these external ketones are the molecules that your body makes for fuel when you are eating a ketogenic diet. By consuming this as a supplement, it can help with entering ketosis faster. They even have some anticancer effects if you are still eating a regular carbohydrate-rich diet. The more you adapt your body to be able to run well on ketones, the more you will be able to starve any cancer cells in your body.

Dmitrieva-Posocco O, Wong AC, Lundgren P, Golos AM, Descamps HC, Dohnalová L, Cramer Z, Tian Y, Yueh B, Eskiocak O, Egervari G, Lan Y, Liu J, Fan J, Kim J, Madhu B, Schneider KM, Khoziainova S, Andreeva N, Wang Q, Li N, Furth EE, Bailis W, Kelsen JR, Hamilton KE, Kaestner KH, Berger SL, Epstein JA, Jain R, Li M, Beyaz S, Lengner CJ, Katona BW, Grivennikov SI, Thaiss CA, Levy M. β-Hydroxybutyrate suppresses colorectal cancer. Nature. 2022 May;605(7908):160-165. doi: 10.1038/s41586-022-04649-6. Epub 2022 Apr 27. PMID: 35477756; PMCID: PMC9448510.

Ferrere G, Tidjani Alou M, Liu P, Goubet AG, Fidelle M, Kepp O, Durand S, Iebba V, Fluckiger A, Daillère R, Thelemaque C, Grajeda-Iglesias C, Alves Costa Silva C, Aprahamian F, Lefevre D, Zhao L, Ryffel B, Colomba E, Arnedos M, Drubay D, Rauber C, Raoult D, Asnicar F, Spector T, Segata N, Derosa L, Kroemer G, Zitvogel L. Ketogenic diet and ketone bodies enhance the anticancer effects of PD-1 blockade. JCI Insight. 2021 Jan 25;6(2):e145207. doi: 10.1172/jci.insight.145207. PMID: 33320838; PMCID: PMC7934884.

Hwang CY, Choe W, Yoon KS, Ha J, Kim SS, Yeo EJ, Kang I. Molecular Mechanisms for Ketone Body Metabolism, Signaling Functions, and Therapeutic Potential in Cancer. Nutrients. 2022 Nov 21;14(22):4932. doi: 10.3390/nu14224932. PMID: 36432618; PMCID: PMC9694619.

-L-

**Lactoferrin-** Lactoferrin is a naturally occurring protein found in human breast milk and other body fluids, including saliva and tears. It has been studied for its potential anti-cancer properties due to its ability to regulate iron metabolism and modulate the immune system. Research has shown that lactoferrin can inhibit the growth and proliferation of cancer cells in vitro and in animal models. It has also been found to have anti-inflammatory effects and can enhance the efficacy of chemotherapy and radiation in cancer treatment.

Cutone A, Rosa L, Ianiro G, Lepanto MS, Bonaccorsi di Patti MC, Valenti P, Musci G. Lactoferrin's Anti-Cancer Properties: Safety, Selectivity, and Wide Range of Action. Biomolecules. 2020 Mar 15;10(3):456. doi: 10.3390/biom10030456. PMID: 32183434; PMCID: PMC7175311.

Rodrigues L, Teixeira J, Schmitt F, Paulsson M, Månsson HL. Lactoferrin and cancer disease prevention. Crit Rev Food Sci Nutr. 2009 Mar;49(3):203-17. doi: 10.1080/10408390701856157. PMID: 19093266.

Pan S, Weng H, Hu G, Wang S, Zhao T, Yao X, Liao L, Zhu X, Ge Y. Lactoferrin may inhibit the development of cancer via its immunostimulatory and immunomodulatory activities (Review). Int J Oncol. 2021 Nov;59(5):85. doi: 10.3892/ijo.2021.5265. Epub 2021 Sep 17. PMID: 34533200.

**Limonene-** is a tiny molecule found in citrus fruits and other plants like mint, juniper, rosemary, and pine needles, that has been studied for its potential cancer-fighting properties. Sweet orange essential oil is one of the richest sources of Limonene. It has been shown to induce apoptosis, or programmed cell death, in cancer cells, as well as inhibit tumor growth and angiogenesis. Studies have also suggested that limonene may have chemopreventive effects, helping to prevent the development of certain types of cancer. Additionally, limonene has been found to have low toxicity and few side effects, making it a promising natural compound for cancer treatment and prevention.

Chebet JJ, Ehiri JE, McClelland DJ, Taren D, Hakim IA. Effect of d-limonene and its derivatives on breast cancer in human trials: a scoping review and narrative synthesis. BMC Cancer. 2021 Aug 6;21(1):902. doi: 10.1186/s12885-021-08639-1. PMID: 34362338; PMCID: PMC8349000.

Crowell PL, Gould MN. Chemoprevention and therapy of cancer by d-limonene. Crit Rev Oncog. 1994;5(1):1-22. doi: 10.1615/critrevoncog.v5.i1.10. PMID: 7948106.

Sun J. D-Limonene: safety and clinical applications. Altern Med Rev. 2007 Sep;12(3):259-64. PMID: 18072821.

Crowell PL, Siar Ayoubi A, Burke YD. Antitumorigenic effects of limonene and perillyl alcohol against pancreatic and breast cancer. Adv Exp Med Biol. 1996;401:131-6. doi: 10.1007/978-1-4613-0399-2_10. PMID: 8886131.

**Low-Dose Naltrexone (LDN)-** is a medication that has been used for the treatment of opioid addiction and alcoholism. However, recent studies have shown its potential in the treatment of cancer. LDN works by binding to opioid receptors in the brain and stimulating the production of endorphins, which can help to reduce inflammation and enhance immune function. This can lead to the suppression of cancer growth and an increase in cancer cell death. LDN is also thought to enhance the effects of chemotherapy and radiation, while reducing their side effects. This must be prescribed by your doctor or licensed naturopath, and is usually custom ordered through a special compounding pharmacy.

Li Z, You Y, Griffin N, Feng J, Shan F. Low-dose naltrexone (LDN): A promising treatment in immune-related diseases and cancer therapy. Int Immunopharmacol. 2018 Aug;61:178-184. doi: 10.1016/j.intimp.2018.05.020. Epub 2018 Jun 7. PMID: 29885638.

Liu WM, Dalgleish AG. Naltrexone at low doses (LDN) and its relevance to cancer therapy. Expert Rev Anticancer Ther. 2022 Mar;22(3):269-274. doi: 10.1080/14737140.2022.2037426. Epub 2022 Feb 7. PMID: 35107043.

Couto RD, Fernandes BJD. Low Doses Naltrexone: The Potential Benefit Effects for its Use in Patients with Cancer. Curr Drug Res Rev. 2021;13(2):86-89. doi: 10.2174/2589977513666210127094222. PMID: 33504322.

**Lumbrokinase**- this is an enzyme that breaks down fibrin and excessive clotting. While it does not have direct anticancer applications, the cancer process creates a higher state of clotting potential or "blood thickness". If you have elevated D-dimer & Fibrinogen labs, this supplement can help to keep the bloodstream flowing properly.

Hu B, Yan Y, Tong F, Xu L, Zhu J, Xu G, Shen R. Lumbrokinase/paclitaxel nanoparticle complex: potential therapeutic applications in bladder cancer. Int J Nanomedicine. 2018 Jun 26;13:3625-3640. doi: 10.2147/IJN.S166438. PMID: 29983558; PMCID: PMC6027826.

**Luteolin**- is a flavonoid compound found in various fruits, vegetables, and herbs including: celery, parsley, sweet & hot peppers, artichokes, and thyme. It exhibits anti-inflammatory and antioxidant properties. Studies suggest that luteolin also has potential in cancer prevention and treatment. Luteolin can induce apoptosis (programmed cell death) in various cancer cells and inhibit cancer cell growth and migration. It may also sensitize cancer cells to chemotherapy and radiation therapy while protecting normal cells. Furthermore, luteolin has shown promise in reducing inflammation associated with cancer and improving immune system function. It lowers VEGF, the protein that stimulates new vessel growth, thus lowering tumor angiogenesis.

Lin Y, Shi R, Wang X, Shen HM. Luteolin, a flavonoid with potential for cancer prevention and therapy. Curr Cancer Drug Targets. 2008 Nov;8(7):634-46. doi: 10.2174/156800908786241050. PMID: 18991571; PMCID: PMC2615542.

Fasoulakis Z, Koutras A, Syllaios A, Schizas D, Garmpis N, Diakosavvas M, Angelou K, Tsatsaris G, Pagkalos A, Ntounis T, Kontomanolis EN. Breast Cancer Apoptosis and the Therapeutic Role of Luteolin. Chirurgia (Bucur). 2021 Mar-Apr;116(2):170-177. doi: 10.21614/chirurgia.116.2.170. PMID: 33950812.

Franza L, Carusi V, Nucera E, Pandolfi F. Luteolin, inflammation and cancer: Special emphasis on gut microbiota. Biofactors. 2021 Mar;47(2):181-189. doi: 10.1002/biof.1710. Epub 2021 Jan 28. PMID: 33507594.

**Lycopene**- is the natural red pigment in tomatoes, pomegranates, watermelons, apricots, and grapefruits. It is most studied to help in prostate cancer. It is better absorbed when eaten with olive oil or other healthy fat sources. This shows the traditional wisdom of homemade Italian tomato sauce made with tomatoes simmered in olive oil. You can supplement with it or increase these natural red foods in your everyday diet.

Moran NE, Thomas-Ahner JM, Wan L, Zuniga KE, Erdman JW, Clinton SK. Tomatoes, Lycopene, and Prostate Cancer: What Have We Learned from Experimental Models? J Nutr. 2022 Jun 9;152(6):1381-1403. doi: 10.1093/jn/nxac066. PMID: 35278075; PMCID: PMC9178968.

Mirahmadi M, Azimi-Hashemi S, Saburi E, Kamali H, Pishbin M, Hadizadeh F. Potential inhibitory effect of lycopene on prostate cancer. Biomed Pharmacother. 2020 Sep;129:110459. doi: 10.1016/j.biopha.2020.110459. Epub 2020 Jun 30. PMID: 32768949.

Chen P, Zhang W, Wang X, Zhao K, Negi DS, Zhuo L, Qi M, Wang X, Zhang X. Lycopene and Risk of Prostate Cancer: A Systematic Review and Meta-Analysis. Medicine (Baltimore). 2015 Aug;94(33):e1260. doi: 10.1097/MD.0000000000001260. PMID: 26287411; PMCID: PMC4616444.

-M-

**Matthias Rath Formula**- Dr Mathias Rath and his team of researchers discovered that the synergistic combination of the nutrients Vitamin-C, Proline, Lysine, and Green Tea extract helped to reduce both heart disease and cancer. One brand option is "Heart Plus" available at https://store.cellnutritionals.com . This nutrient combination helps to block MMP enzymes that dissolve collagen and allow cancers to spread. It also builds collagen and strengthens arteries.

Roomi MW, Ivanov V, Kalinovsky T, Niedzwiecki A, Rath M. Antitumor effect of ascorbic acid, lysine, proline, arginine, and green tea extract on bladder cancer cell line T-24. Int J Urol. 2006 Apr;13(4):415-9. doi: 10.1111/j.1442-2042.2006.01309.x. PMID: 16734861.

Roomi MW, Ivanov V, Kalinovsky T, Niedzwiecki A, Rath M. Inhibition of matrix metalloproteinase-2 secretion and invasion by human ovarian cancer cell line SK-OV-3 with lysine, proline, arginine, ascorbic acid and green tea extract. J Obstet Gynaecol Res. 2006 Apr;32(2):148-54. doi: 10.1111/j.1447-0756.2006.00389.x. PMID: 16594917.

Roomi MW, Ivanov V, Kalinovsky T, Niedzwiecki A, Rath M. Suppression of human cervical cancer cell lines Hela and DoTc2 4510 by a mixture of lysine, proline, ascorbic acid, and green tea extract. Int J Gynecol Cancer. 2006 May-Jun;16(3):1241-7. doi: 10.1111/j.1525-1438.2006.00545.x. PMID: 16803512.

**Medium Chain Triglyceride (MCT) Oil (Liquid or Powder)-** has been suggested as complementary therapy for cancer treatment and prevention due to its unique properties. MCTs are rapidly metabolized by the body and are a source of readily available energy. Studies have shown that MCT oil can help reduce body weight and body fat, both of which are risk factors for cancer development. Additionally, MCT oil has been found to have anti-inflammatory and antioxidant effects, which may also be beneficial for cancer prevention. It is a helpful supplement to a ketogenic diet for quick energy throughout the day.

Nebeling LC, Lerner E. Implementing a ketogenic diet based on medium-chain triglyceride oil in pediatric patients with cancer. J Am Diet Assoc. 1995 Jun;95(6):693-7. doi: 10.1016/S0002-8223(95)00189-1. PMID: 7759747.

Cury-Boaventura MF, Torrinhas RS, de Godoy AB, Curi R, Waitzberg DL. Human leukocyte death after a preoperative infusion of medium/long-chain triglyceride and fish oil parenteral emulsions: a randomized study in gastrointestinal cancer patients. JPEN J Parenter Enteral Nutr. 2012 Nov;36(6):677-84. doi: 10.1177/0148607111432759. Epub 2012 Jan 26. PMID: 22282868.

**Melatonin-** is the famous hormone produced by the pineal gland that regulates sleep-wake cycles. In recent years, it has gained attention for its role in Naturopathic cancer treatment and prevention. Studies have shown that melatonin can help inhibit the growth of cancer cells by promoting apoptosis (programmed cell death) and reducing the formation of new blood vessels that support tumor growth. It also enhances the effectiveness of chemotherapy drugs and reduces their side effects. Additionally, research suggests that melatonin can help prevent cancer by acting as an antioxidant and protecting cells from DNA damage caused by free radicals. 20 mg at bedtime is the most common dose for cancer treatment.

Talib WH. Melatonin and Cancer Hallmarks. Molecules. 2018 Feb 26;23(3):518. doi: 10.3390/molecules23030518. PMID: 29495398; PMCID: PMC6017729.

Li Y, Li S, Zhou Y, Meng X, Zhang JJ, Xu DP, Li HB. Melatonin for the prevention and treatment of cancer. Oncotarget. 2017 Jun 13;8(24):39896-39921. doi: 10.18632/oncotarget.16379. PMID: 28415828; PMCID: PMC5503661.

Talib WH, Alsayed AR, Abuawad A, Daoud S, Mahmod AI. Melatonin in Cancer Treatment: Current Knowledge and Future Opportunities. Molecules. 2021 Apr 25;26(9):2506. doi: 10.3390/molecules26092506. PMID: 33923028; PMCID: PMC8123278.

**Met-Enkephalin-** is an endogenous opioid peptide that has been shown to have anti-cancer properties. Studies have demonstrated that it can inhibit tumor growth and induce apoptosis in various cancer cell lines. Met-enkephalin has also been shown to enhance the effects of

chemotherapy and radiation, making it a promising therapeutic agent for cancer treatment. Additionally, met-enkephalin has been found to have immunomodulatory effects, which improves the body's ability to fight cancer.

Zhao D, Plotnikoff N, Griffin N, Song T, Shan F. Methionine enkephalin, its role in immunoregulation and cancer therapy. Int Immunopharmacol. 2016 Aug;37:59-64. doi: 10.1016/j.intimp.2016.02.015. Epub 2016 Feb 24. PMID: 26927200.

Zhang S, Liu N, Ma M, Huang H, Handley M, Bai X, Shan F. Methionine enkephalin (MENK) suppresses lung cancer by regulating the Bcl-2/Bax/caspase-3 signaling pathway and enhancing natural killer cell-driven tumor immunity. Int Immunopharmacol. 2021 Sep;98:107837. doi: 10.1016/j.intimp.2021.107837. Epub 2021 Jun 8. PMID: 34116288.

Kajdaniuk D, Marek B, Swietochowska E, Ciesielska-Kopacz N, Buntner B. Is positive correlation between cortisol and met-enkephalin concentration in blood of women with breast cancer a reaction to stress before chemotherapy administration? Pathophysiology. 2000 Apr;7(1):47-51. doi: 10.1016/s0928-4680(00)00028-6. PMID: 10825685.

**Metformin**- is a widely used medication for type 2 diabetes, but it has also shown potential for cancer treatment and prevention. Studies suggest that Metformin can reduce the risk of various cancers, including breast, colon, and pancreatic cancers. It has also shown to improve the effectiveness of chemotherapy in cancer treatment by inhibiting cancer cell growth and inducing cell death. Additionally, Metformin has been shown to reduce insulin resistance and inflammation, which are factors that contribute to cancer development.

Podhorecka M, Ibanez B, Dmoszyńska A. Metformin - its potential anti-cancer and anti-aging effects. Postepy Hig Med Dosw (Online). 2017 Mar 2;71(0):170-175. doi: 10.5604/01.3001.0010.3801. PMID: 28258677.

Vallianou NG, Evangelopoulos A, Kazazis C. Metformin and cancer. Rev Diabet Stud. 2013 Winter;10(4):228-35. doi: 10.1900/RDS.2013.10.228. Epub 2014 Feb 10. PMID: 24841876; PMCID: PMC4160009.

Morales DR, Morris AD. Metformin in cancer treatment and prevention. Annu Rev Med. 2015;66:17-29. doi: 10.1146/annurev-med-062613-093128. Epub 2014 Nov 6. PMID: 25386929.

**Modified Citrus Pectin (MCP)-** is a fiber derived from the peels of citrus fruits. It has been extensively studied for its anti-cancer properties. MCP has been shown to inhibit cancer cell growth, prevent the formation of new blood vessels that tumors rely on for their growth, modulate the immune system, and improve the efficacy of chemotherapy drugs. It blocks a protein called galectin-3 that increases the cancer process. Additionally, MCP has been shown to improve immune function, which is important in cancer prevention and treatment. MCP may also have a role in preventing cancer metastasis, as it has been shown to inhibit cancer cell adhesion and migration.

Keizman D, Frenkel M, Peer A, Kushnir I, Rosenbaum E, Sarid D, Leibovitch I, Mano R, Yossepowitch O, Margel D, Wolf I, Geva R, Dresler H, Rouvinov K, Rapoport N, Eliaz I. Modified Citrus Pectin Treatment in Non-Metastatic Biochemically Relapsed Prostate Cancer: Results of a Prospective Phase II Study. Nutrients. 2021 Nov 28;13(12):4295. doi: 10.3390/nu13124295. PMID: 34959847; PMCID: PMC8706421.

Wang L, Zhao L, Gong FL, Sun C, Du DD, Yang XX, Guo XL. Modified citrus pectin inhibits breast cancer development in mice by targeting tumor-associated macrophage survival and polarization in hypoxic microenvironment. Acta Pharmacol Sin. 2022 Jun;43(6):1556-1567. doi: 10.1038/s41401-021-00748-8. Epub 2021 Aug 30. PMID: 34462562; PMCID: PMC9160294.

-N-

**Nattokinase-** is a proteolytic enzyme derived from the traditional Japanese food natto. Studies have shown that nattokinase has anticancer properties and may help to prevent the growth and spread of cancer cells. This may be due to its ability to inhibit angiogenesis, the process by which tumors develop new blood vessels to feed themselves. Additionally, nattokinase has been shown to have anti-inflammatory effects, which may also contribute to its potential anticancer activity.

Zhang Y, Pei P, Zhou H, Xie Y, Yang S, Shen W, Hu L, Zhang Y, Liu T, Yang K. Nattokinase-Mediated Regulation of Tumor Physical Microenvironment to Enhance Chemotherapy, Radiotherapy, and CAR-T Therapy of Solid Tumor. ACS Nano. 2023 Apr 25;17(8):7475-7486. doi: 10.1021/acsnano.2c12463. Epub 2023 Apr 14. PMID: 37057972.

Kou Y, Feng R, Chen J, Duan L, Wang S, Hu Y, Zhang N, Wang T, Deng Y, Song Y. Development of a nattokinase-polysialic acid complex for advanced tumor treatment. Eur J Pharm Sci. 2020 Mar 30;145:105241. doi: 10.1016/j.ejps.2020.105241. Epub 2020 Jan 28. PMID: 32001345.

**Nicotinamide Adenine Dinucleotide and Hydrogen (NADH)**- is a coenzyme that plays a crucial role in the production of energy in cells. It has been studied for its potential in cancer treatment and prevention due to its ability to improve cellular metabolism and immune function. NADH has been shown to reduce oxidative stress and inflammation, two factors that can contribute to the development and progression of cancer. Studies have also suggested that NADH may enhance the effectiveness of chemotherapy and radiation therapy in cancer patients.

Pramono AA, Rather GM, Herman H, Lestari K, Bertino JR. NAD- and NADPH-Contributing Enzymes as Therapeutic Targets in Cancer: An Overview. Biomolecules. 2020 Feb 26;10(3):358. doi: 10.3390/biom10030358. PMID: 32111066; PMCID: PMC7175141.

Weiss-Sadan T, Ge M, Hayashi M, Gohar M, Yao CH, de Groot A, Harry S, Carlin A, Fischer H, Shi L, Wei TY, Adelmann CH, Wolf K, Vornbäumen T, Dürr BR, Takahashi M, Richter M, Zhang J, Yang TY, Vijay V, Fisher DE, Hata AN, Haigis MC, Mostoslavsky R, Bardeesy N, Papagiannakopoulos T, Bar-Peled L. NRF2 activation induces NADH-reductive stress, providing a metabolic vulnerability in lung cancer. Cell Metab. 2023 Mar 7;35(3):487-503.e7. doi: 10.1016/j.cmet.2023.01.012. Epub 2023 Feb 24. Erratum in: Cell Metab. 2023 Apr 4;35(4):722. PMID: 36841242; PMCID: PMC9998367.

-P-

**Pancreatic Enzymes**- enzyme therapy for cancer was first pioneered by Dr John Beard about 100 years ago. Later, Dr William Kelley, Dr Nicholas Gonzalez, and Dr Linda Issacs have continued studying and using this powerful therapy. Enzymes such as trypsin and chymotrypsin are produced by the pancreas to help break down and digest food in the small intestine. These enzymes can also be used as a complementary therapy in cancer treatment, particularly pancreatic cancer. They are believed to have antitumor properties that can help break down the protective coating surrounding cancer cells, making them more vulnerable to the immune system and conventional therapies. Pancreatic enzymes have also been shown to reduce inflammation and improve overall digestive health, which can be particularly important for cancer patients who may experience digestive issues due to treatments such as chemotherapy. One recommended brand is called Wobe-Mucos E or Wobenzyme.

Isaacs LL. Pancreatic Proteolytic Enzymes and Cancer: New Support for an Old Theory. Integr Cancer Ther. 2022 Jan-Dec;21:15347354221096077. doi: 10.1177/15347354221096077. PMID: 35514109; PMCID: PMC9083047.

Moss RW. Enzymes, trophoblasts, and cancer: the afterlife of an idea (1924-2008). Integr Cancer Ther. 2008 Dec;7(4):262-75. doi: 10.1177/1534735408326172. PMID: 19116222.

Popiela T, Kulig J, Kłek S, Wachol D, Bock PR, Hanisch J. Double-blind pilot-study on the efficacy of enzyme therapy in advanced colorectal cancer. Przegl Lek. 2000;57 Suppl 5:142. PMID: 11202281.

**pH Balance (Acid/Base)**- pH balance is the measure of the acidity or alkalinity in the body. On the pH scale, 1 is extremely acidic, 14 is the ultimate alkaline, and 7 is neutral. The body's natural pH is slightly alkaline, around 7.4. A diet that is high in acidic foods can lead to a drop in pH, which may contribute to the growth and spread of cancer cells. Cancer cells also create their own acidic local environment due to their unique metabolism. The more acidic the tissue is around a tumor, the more it can evade the immune system, grow more rapidly, and spread throughout the body. Maintaining a healthy pH balance through a diet rich in alkaline foods, such as fruits, vegetables, greens, nuts, and seeds can help prevent cancer and improve cancer treatment outcomes. Supplemental potassium citrate and potassium bicarbonate can also be helpful to lower the overall acidity of the body. If you supplement with alkalizing pills or powders, do it between meals to avoid neutralizing your stomach acid that is needed for digestion. You can purchase pH testing strips on Amazon or other online stores for urine or saliva and monitor your own ph levels at home. Aim for saliva and first-morning urine pH levels between 7 - 7.4

Ibrahim-Hashim A, Estrella V. Acidosis and cancer: from mechanism to neutralization. Cancer Metastasis Rev. 2019 Jun;38(1-2):149-155. doi: 10.1007/s10555-019-09787-4. PMID: 30806853; PMCID: PMC6625834.

Becker HM, Deitmer JW. Transport Metabolons and Acid/Base Balance in Tumor Cells. Cancers (Basel). 2020 Apr 7;12(4):899. doi: 10.3390/cancers12040899. PMID: 32272695; PMCID: PMC7226098.

Ando H, Eshima K, Ishida T. Neutralization of Acidic Tumor Microenvironment (TME) with Daily Oral Dosing of Sodium Potassium Citrate (K/Na Citrate) Increases Therapeutic Effect of Anti-cancer Agent in Pancreatic Cancer Xenograft Mice Model. Biol Pharm Bull. 2021;44(2):266-270. doi: 10.1248/bpb.b20-00825. PMID: 33518679.

**PNC-27**- is a peptide consisting of 27 amino acids, which is derived from human pancreatic ribonuclease. Research has shown that PNC-27 has anticancer properties and can selectively target cancer cells by binding to their membranes. When PNC-27 enters the cancer cell, it induces apoptosis or programmed cell death, leading to the destruction of the cancer cell. Studies have also demonstrated that PNC-27 can enhance the effectiveness of chemotherapy and radiation, making conventional cancer treatments more effective.

Alagkiozidis I, Gorelick C, Shah T, Chen YA, Gupta V, Stefanov D, Amarnani A, Lee YC, Abulafia O, Sarafraz-Yazdi E, Michl J. Synergy between Paclitaxel and Anti-Cancer Peptide PNC-27 in the Treatment of Ovarian Cancer. Ann Clin Lab Sci. 2017 May;47(3):271-281. PMID: 28667027.

Sookraj KA, Bowne WB, Adler V, Sarafraz-Yazdi E, Michl J, Pincus MR. The anti-cancer peptide, PNC-27, induces tumor cell lysis as the intact peptide. Cancer Chemother Pharmacol. 2010 Jul;66(2):325-31. doi: 10.1007/s00280-009-1166-7. Epub 2010 Feb 25. PMID: 20182728.

**Poly MVA**- is a dietary supplement that contains palladium and other vitamins and minerals. It has potential as a cancer treatment due to its ability to enhance the body's natural antioxidant system, stimulate the immune system, and promote DNA repair. Some studies have shown that Poly MVA may be effective in reducing tumor growth and improving quality of life in cancer patients. It has been most studied for its use as an adjunctive with radiation therapy.

Veena RK, Ajith TA, Janardhanan KK, Antonawich F. Antitumor Effects of Palladium-α-Lipoic Acid Complex Formulation as an Adjunct in Radiotherapy. J Environ Pathol Toxicol Oncol. 2016;35(4):333-342. doi: 10.1615/JEnvironPatholToxicolOncol.2016016640. PMID: 27992313.

Ramachandran L, Krishnan CV, Nair CK. Radioprotection by alpha-lipoic acid palladium complex formulation (POLY-MVA) in mice. Cancer Biother Radiopharm. 2010 Aug;25(4):395-9. doi: 10.1089/cbr.2009.0744. PMID: 20701542.

**Probiotics**- The field of probiotics is a mind-bogglingly vast area of medical research. So it is difficult for doctors and researchers to ever keep up to date with the studies on the microbiome. Probiotics and cancer is a very complex and ever-developing area of research, however one key molecule we know about that links the two is butyrate. Butyrate is a short-chain fatty acid that is produced in the gut by many species of probiotic bacteria. Butyrate is also available as an oral supplement or as a rectal enema.

Butyrate has been shown to support cancer treatments in several ways:

**Anti-inflammatory properties**- Butyrate has anti-inflammatory properties that can help reduce inflammation in the body. Inflammation has been linked to the development of cancer and can also make cancer treatment less effective. By reducing inflammation, butyrate can help support cancer treatments.

**Anti-tumor properties**- Butyrate has been shown to have anti-tumor properties, meaning it can help inhibit the growth of cancer cells. This can be particularly helpful in supporting cancer treatments by reducing the spread of cancer.

**Enhances immune function**- Butyrate has been shown to enhance immune function, which can help the body fight cancer. A strong immune system is important in fighting cancer, and butyrate can help support this function.

**Improves gut health**- Butyrate is produced by the gut microbiota through fermentation of dietary fiber. It has been shown to improve gut health and reduce the risk of gut disorders. This can be particularly helpful in supporting cancer treatments, as some cancer treatments can damage the gut microbiota.

**Enhances chemotherapy effectiveness**- Butyrate has been shown to enhance the effectiveness of chemotherapy in some studies. By improving the effectiveness of chemotherapy, butyrate can help support cancer treatments.

Eslami M, Yousefi B, Kokhaei P, Hemati M, Nejad ZR, Arabkari V, Namdar A. Importance of probiotics in the prevention and treatment of colorectal cancer. J Cell Physiol. 2019 Aug;234(10):17127-17143. doi: 10.1002/jcp.28473. Epub 2019 Mar 25. PMID: 30912128.

Legesse Bedada T, Feto TK, Awoke KS, Garedew AD, Yifat FT, Birri DJ. Probiotics for cancer alternative prevention and treatment. Biomed Pharmacother. 2020 Sep;129:110409. doi: 10.1016/j.biopha.2020.110409. Epub 2020 Jun 18. PMID: 32563987.

Badgeley A, Anwar H, Modi K, Murphy P, Lakshmikuttyamma A. Effect of probiotics and gut microbiota on anti-cancer drugs: Mechanistic perspectives. Biochim Biophys Acta Rev Cancer. 2021 Jan;1875(1):188494. doi: 10.1016/j.bbcan.2020.188494. Epub 2020 Dec 17. PMID: 33346129.

The following probiotic strains are known to help produce butyrate in the gut.

**Faecalibacterium prausnitzii**- This probiotic strain is known to be a major producer of butyrate in the gut. It is also associated with anti-inflammatory properties and has been shown to be reduced in individuals with gut disorders.

Dikeocha IJ, Al-Kabsi AM, Chiu HT, Alshawsh MA. *Faecalibacterium prausnitzii* Ameliorates Colorectal Tumorigenesis and Suppresses Proliferation of HCT116 Colorectal Cancer Cells. Biomedicines. 2022 May 13;10(5):1128. doi: 10.3390/biomedicines10051128. PMID: 35625865; PMCID: PMC9138996.

**Eubacterium rectale**- This strain is also known to be a significant producer of butyrate in the gut. It has been shown to be decreased in individuals with inflammatory bowel disease.

Wang Y, Wan X, Wu X, Zhang C, Liu J, Hou S. Eubacterium rectale contributes to colorectal cancer initiation via promoting colitis. Gut Pathog. 2021 Jan 12;13(1):2. doi: 10.1186/s13099-020-00396-z. PMID: 33436075; PMCID: PMC7805161.

**Roseburia spp**- This group of probiotic strains is known to be involved in butyrate production and has been associated with improved gut health.

Tamanai-Shacoori Z, Smida I, Bousarghin L, Loreal O, Meuric V, Fong SB, Bonnaure-Mallet M, Jolivet-Gougeon A. Roseburia spp.: a marker of health? Future Microbiol. 2017 Feb;12:157-170. doi: 10.2217/fmb-2016-0130. PMID: 28139139.

Gui Q, Li H, Wang A, Zhao X, Tan Z, Chen L, Xu K, Xiao C. The association between gut butyrate-producing bacteria and non-small-cell lung cancer. J Clin Lab Anal. 2020 Aug;34(8):e23318. doi: 10.1002/jcla.23318. Epub 2020 Mar 29. PMID: 32227387; PMCID: PMC7439349.

**Bifidobacterium lactis**- This probiotic strain has been shown to increase butyrate production in the gut and is commonly used in probiotic supplements.

Bozkurt HS, Quigley EM, Kara B. *Bifidobacterium animalis* subspecies *lactis* engineered to produce mycosporin-like amino acids in colorectal cancer prevention. SAGE Open Med. 2019 Jan 22;7:2050312119825784. doi: 10.1177/2050312119825784. PMID: 30719295; PMCID: PMC6348500.

**Lactobacillus plantarum**- This strain has been shown to increase butyrate production and improve gut health in animal studies.

Sharifi E, Yazdani Z, Najafi M, Hosseini-Khah Z, Jafarpour A, Rafiei A. The combined effect of fish oil containing Omega-3 fatty acids and *Lactobacillus plantarum* on colorectal cancer. Food Sci Nutr. 2022 Sep 28;10(12):4411-4418. doi: 10.1002/fsn3.3037. PMID: 36514755; PMCID: PMC9731559.

Common probiotic strains that have been shown to be helpful in cancer treatment include:

**Lactobacillus acidophilus**- This probiotic strain has been shown to enhance the immune system and reduce inflammation, which can be helpful in supporting cancer treatment.

Yue Y, Wang S, Shi J, Xie Q, Li N, Guan J, Evivie SE, Liu F, Li B, Huo G. Effects of *Lactobacillus acidophilus* KLDS1.0901 on Proliferation and Apoptosis of Colon Cancer Cells. Front Microbiol. 2022 Feb 11;12:788040. doi: 10.3389/fmicb.2021.788040. PMID: 35250903; PMCID: PMC8895954.

Onur E, Gökmen GG, Nalbantsoy A, Kışla D. Investigation of the supportive therapy potential of propolis extract and Lactobacillus acidophilus LA-5 milk combination against breast cancer in mice. Cytokine. 2022 Jan;149:155743. doi: 10.1016/j.cyto.2021.155743. Epub 2021 Oct 15. PMID: 34662821.

**Bifidobacterium bifidum**- This probiotic strain has been shown to reduce inflammation and support the immune system, which can help the body fight cancer.

Lee SH, Cho SY, Yoon Y, Park C, Sohn J, Jeong JJ, Jeon BN, Jang M, An C, Lee S, Kim YY, Kim G, Kim S, Kim Y, Lee GB, Lee EJ, Kim SG, Kim HS, Kim Y, Kim H, Yang HS, Kim S, Kim S, Chung H, Moon MH, Nam MH, Kwon JY, Won S, Park JS, Weinstock GM, Lee C, Yoon KW,

Park H. Bifidobacterium bifidum strains synergize with immune checkpoint inhibitors to reduce tumour burden in mice. Nat Microbiol. 2021 Mar;6(3):277-288. doi: 10.1038/s41564-020-00831-6. Epub 2021 Jan 11. PMID: 33432149.

Benito I, Encío IJ, Milagro FI, Alfaro M, Martínez-Peñuela A, Barajas M, Marzo F. Microencapsulated *Bifidobacterium bifidum* and *Lactobacillus gasseri* in Combination with Quercetin Inhibit Colorectal Cancer Development in ApcMin/+ Mice. Int J Mol Sci. 2021 May 5;22(9):4906. doi: 10.3390/ijms22094906. PMID: 34063173; PMCID: PMC8124226.

Reghu S, Miyako E. Nanoengineered *Bifidobacterium bifidum* with Optical Activity for Photothermal Cancer Immunotheranostics. Nano Lett. 2022 Mar 9;22(5):1880-1888. doi: 10.1021/acs.nanolett.1c04037. Epub 2022 Feb 18. PMID: 35179380.

**Lactobacillus rhamnosus GG**- This strain has been shown to reduce inflammation, enhance immune function, and improve gut health. It has been studied for its potential to support cancer treatment and improve quality of life in cancer patients.

Banna GL, Torino F, Marletta F, Santagati M, Salemi R, Cannarozzo E, Falzone L, Ferraù F, Libra M. *Lactobacillus rhamnosus* GG: An Overview to Explore the Rationale of Its Use in Cancer. Front Pharmacol. 2017 Sep 1;8:603. doi: 10.3389/fphar.2017.00603. PMID: 28919861; PMCID: PMC5585742.

Salemi R, Vivarelli S, Ricci D, Scillato M, Santagati M, Gattuso G, Falzone L, Libra M. Lactobacillus rhamnosus GG cell-free supernatant as a novel anti-cancer adjuvant. J Transl Med. 2023 Mar 14;21(1):195. doi: 10.1186/s12967-023-04036-3. PMID: 36918929; PMCID: PMC10015962.

Keyhani G, Mahmoodzadeh Hosseini H, Salimi A. Effect of extracellular vesicles of *Lactobacillus rhamnosus* GG on the expression of CEA gene and protein released by colorectal cancer cells. Iran J Microbiol. 2022 Feb;14(1):90-96. doi: 10.18502/ijm.v14i1.8809. PMID: 35664711; PMCID: PMC9085540.

**Streptococcus thermophilus**-This probiotic strain has been studied for its potential to support cancer treatment by enhancing immune function and reducing inflammation.

Tarrah A, de Castilhos J, Rossi RC, Duarte VDS, Ziegler DR, Corich V, Giacomini A. *In vitro* Probiotic Potential and Anti-cancer Activity of Newly Isolated Folate-Producing *Streptococcus thermophilus* Strains. Front Microbiol. 2018 Sep 19;9:2214. doi: 10.3389/fmicb.2018.02214. PMID: 30283428; PMCID: PMC6156529.

Hadad SE, Alsolami M, Aldahlawi A, Alrahimi J, Basingab F, Hassoubah S, Alothaid H. *In vivo* evidence: Repression of mucosal immune responses in mice with colon cancer following sustained administration of *Streptococcus thermophiles*. Saudi J Biol Sci. 2021

Aug;28(8):4751-4761. doi: 10.1016/j.sjbs.2021.04.090. Epub 2021 May 6. PMID: 34354463; PMCID: PMC8324971.

**Saccharomyces boulardii**- This probiotic yeast strain has been shown to improve gut health and reduce inflammation. It has been studied for its potential to support cancer treatment and reduce the side effects of chemotherapy and radiation therapy.

Pakbin B, Allahyari S, Dibazar SP, Peymani A, Haghverdi MK, Taherkhani K, Javadi M, Mahmoudi R. Anticancer Properties of Saccharomyces boulardii Metabolite Against Colon Cancer Cells. Probiotics Antimicrob Proteins. 2022 Dec 22. doi: 10.1007/s12602-022-10030-w. Epub ahead of print. PMID: 36547769.

Pakbin B, Pishkhan Dibazar S, Allahyari S, Javadi M, Farasat A, Darzi S. Probiotic *Saccharomyces cerevisiae* var. *boulardii* supernatant inhibits survivin gene expression and induces apoptosis in human gastric cancer cells. Food Sci Nutr. 2020 Nov 29;9(2):692-700. doi: 10.1002/fsn3.2032. PMID: 33598154; PMCID: PMC7866606.

Pakbin B, Dibazar SP, Allahyari S, Javadi M, Amani Z, Farasat A, Darzi S. Anticancer Properties of Probiotic Saccharomyces boulardii Supernatant on Human Breast Cancer Cells. Probiotics Antimicrob Proteins. 2022 Dec;14(6):1130-1138. doi: 10.1007/s12602-021-09756-w. Epub 2022 Jan 30. PMID: 35094296.

**Propolis**- This is a resin produced by bees in their hives. It is a powerful antibacterial, antiviral, antifungal, and contains at least two known anti-cancer compounds: caffeic acid phenethyl ester (CAPE) and apigenin. Propolis has been shown to inhibit the growth and proliferation of cancer cells and induce apoptosis, or programmed cell death, in various types of cancer. Propolis has also been reported to have anti-inflammatory and immunomodulatory effects, which may contribute to its anti-cancer properties. Bee propolis is available in jars like honey or in supplemental capsules.

Forma E, Bryś M. Anticancer Activity of Propolis and Its Compounds. Nutrients. 2021 Jul 28;13(8):2594. doi: 10.3390/nu13082594. PMID: 34444754; PMCID: PMC8399583.

Oršolić N, Jazvinšćak Jembrek M. Molecular and Cellular Mechanisms of Propolis and Its Polyphenolic Compounds against Cancer. Int J Mol Sci. 2022 Sep 9;23(18):10479. doi: 10.3390/ijms231810479. PMID: 36142391; PMCID: PMC9499605.

Masadah R, Ikram D, Rauf S. Effects of propolis and its bioactive components on breast cancer cell pathways and the molecular mechanisms involved. Breast Dis. 2021;40(S1):S15-S25. doi: 10.3233/BD-219003. PMID: 34057114.

**Pterostilbene-** is a compound related to resveratrol found in plants such as blueberries, grapes, and Pterocarpus marsupium (Kino tree) that has been studied for its potential benefits in cancer treatment and prevention. Pterostilbene is known to activate sirtuins, enzymes that play a role in DNA repair, metabolism, and potentially extending lifespan. In lab studies, pterostilbene has been shown to inhibit the growth of various types of cancer cells, including breast, colon, lung, and liver cancer cells. It may also work by reducing inflammation, oxidative stress, and DNA damage, which are all factors that contribute to cancer development. Pterostilbene may also enhance the effectiveness of certain cancer treatments, such as radiation therapy, by sensitizing cancer cells to the treatment. It is also being studied for longevity and improving brain health.

Obrador E, Salvador-Palmer R, Jihad-Jebbar A, López-Blanch R, Dellinger TH, Dellinger RW, Estrela JM. Pterostilbene in Cancer Therapy. Antioxidants (Basel). 2021 Mar 21;10(3):492. doi: 10.3390/antiox10030492. PMID: 33801098; PMCID: PMC8004113.

McCormack D, McFadden D. Pterostilbene and cancer: current review. J Surg Res. 2012 Apr;173(2):e53-61. doi: 10.1016/j.jss.2011.09.054. Epub 2011 Oct 21. PMID: 22099605.

Chen RJ, Kuo HC, Cheng LH, Lee YH, Chang WT, Wang BJ, Wang YJ, Cheng HC. Apoptotic and Nonapoptotic Activities of Pterostilbene against Cancer. Int J Mol Sci. 2018 Jan 18;19(1):287. doi: 10.3390/ijms19010287. PMID: 29346311; PMCID: PMC5796233.

-Q-

**Quercetin-** is a flavonoid commonly found in foods and beverages such as onions, apples, berries, and tea. It has been shown to have anti-inflammatory, antioxidant, antihistamine, and anti-cancer properties. Studies have demonstrated that quercetin can inhibit cancer cell growth and induce apoptosis, or programmed cell death, in various cancer types including breast, colon, prostate, and lung cancer. Quercetin may also enhance the effectiveness of chemotherapy and radiation therapy by increasing cancer cell sensitivity to treatment while protecting healthy cells. Additionally, quercetin's anti-inflammatory properties may help reduce cancer-related inflammation and the risk of cancer development.

Tang SM, Deng XT, Zhou J, Li QP, Ge XX, Miao L. Pharmacological basis and new insights of quercetin action in respect to its anti-cancer effects. Biomed Pharmacother. 2020 Jan;121:109604. doi: 10.1016/j.biopha.2019.109604. Epub 2019 Nov 13. PMID: 31733570.

Reyes-Farias M, Carrasco-Pozo C. The Anti-Cancer Effect of Quercetin: Molecular Implications in Cancer Metabolism. Int J Mol Sci. 2019 Jun 28;20(13):3177. doi: 10.3390/ijms20133177. PMID: 31261749; PMCID: PMC6651418.

Wang ZX, Ma J, Li XY, Wu Y, Shi H, Chen Y, Lu G, Shen HM, Lu GD, Zhou J. Quercetin induces p53-independent cancer cell death through lysosome activation by the transcription factor EB and Reactive Oxygen Species-dependent ferroptosis. Br J Pharmacol. 2021 Mar;178(5):1133-1148. doi: 10.1111/bph.15350. Epub 2021 Feb 2. PMID: 33347603.

-R-

**Resveratrol-** is a naturally occurring polyphenol most often found in red grape skins and Japanese knotweed that has been found to have anticancer properties. It has been shown to inhibit cancer cell growth and promote apoptosis, or programmed cell death. Resveratrol has also been found to have anti-inflammatory effects, which can help prevent cancer by reducing inflammation in the body. Additionally, resveratrol has been shown to have antioxidant properties, which can help protect cells from damage and may help prevent cancer from developing. Overall, research suggests that resveratrol is a promising agent in cancer prevention and treatment as well as human longevity.

Ren B, Kwah MX, Liu C, Ma Z, Shanmugam MK, Ding L, Xiang X, Ho PC, Wang L, Ong PS, Goh BC. Resveratrol for cancer therapy: Challenges and future perspectives. Cancer Lett. 2021 Sep 1;515:63-72. doi: 10.1016/j.canlet.2021.05.001. Epub 2021 May 28. PMID: 34052324.

Zaffaroni N, Beretta GL. Resveratrol and Prostate Cancer: The Power of Phytochemicals. Curr Med Chem. 2021;28(24):4845-4862. doi: 10.2174/0929867328666201228124038. PMID: 33371831.

Vernousfaderani EK, Akhtari N, Rezaei S, Rezaee Y, Shiranirad S, Mashhadi M, Hashemi A, Khankandi HP, Behzad S. Resveratrol and Colorectal Cancer: A Molecular Approach to Clinical Researches. Curr Top Med Chem. 2021;21(29):2634-2646. doi: 10.2174/1568026621666211105093658. PMID: 34749615

-S-

**Salicinium-** Orasal is the oral version, and Salicinium is an IV or injected version. This is a compound that has been studied to have anti-cancer properties. It has been used by many integrative cancer clinics around the world. It is thought to work by selectively targeting cancer cells, inducing apoptosis and inhibiting angiogenesis, and suppressing the activity of cancer-promoting enzymes. It is compatible with most chemotherapies and helps destroy the protective cloak of protein around cancer cells. It only affects anaerobic cells like cancer cells, so it is a very targeted treatment. It helps macrophage immune cells to recognize cancer, and it slows the production of nagalase and lactate. It affects circulating tumor cells first, and stimulates the body's natural GcMAF (macrophage activating factor). While no scientific papers on this substance could be found on Pubmed.gov, it has a history of safe and effective use among many cancer-care clinics.

**Salvestrols-** This is another name for the powerful plant chemicals that are made as defenses against predators, mold, or ultraviolet light in many different plants and fruits. Phytoalexins such as resveratrol and pterostilbene are in this category. There is a supplement called Salvestrol 2000, that is reported to contain a large amount of these healthy plant molecules.

Yamashita N, Taga C, Ozawa M, Kanno Y, Sanada N, Kizu R. Camalexin, an indole phytoalexin, inhibits cell proliferation, migration, and mammosphere formation in breast cancer cells via the aryl hydrocarbon receptor. J Nat Med. 2022 Jan;76(1):110-118. doi: 10.1007/s11418-021-01560-8. Epub 2021 Aug 31. PMID: 34463909.

Jiang Z, Chen K, Cheng L, Yan B, Qian W, Cao J, Li J, Wu E, Ma Q, Yang W. Resveratrol and cancer treatment: updates. Ann N Y Acad Sci. 2017 Sep;1403(1):59-69. doi: 10.1111/nyas.13466. PMID: 28945938.

Navarro-Orcajada S, Vidal-Sánchez FJ, Conesa I, Escribano-Naharro F, Matencio A, López-Nicolás JM. Antiproliferative Effects in Colorectal Cancer and Stabilisation in Cyclodextrins of the Phytoalexin Isorhapontigenin. Biomedicines. 2023 Nov 10;11(11):3023. doi: 10.3390/biomedicines11113023. PMID: 38002023.

**Scutellarein-** is a flavone found in several plants (Chinese skullcap, western skullcap, mint, rosemary, parsley, blueberries, and cherries) that exhibits anti-cancer properties. It has been shown to induce apoptosis, or programmed cell death, in various cancer cell lines, including lung, breast, and cervical cancer. Scutellarein has also been found to inhibit cancer cell proliferation, migration, and invasion, as well as angiogenesis. These effects are thought to be mediated through various signaling pathways, including the PI3K/Akt and MAPK pathways.

Shi X, Chen G, Liu X, Qiu Y, Yang S, Zhang Y, Fang X, Zhang C, Liu X. Scutellarein inhibits cancer cell metastasis in vitro and attenuates the development of fibrosarcoma in vivo. Int J Mol Med. 2015 Jan;35(1):31-8. doi: 10.3892/ijmm.2014.1997. Epub 2014 Nov 12. PMID: 25394920; PMCID: PMC4249742.

Gowda Saralamma VV, Lee HJ, Raha S, Lee WS, Kim EH, Lee SJ, Heo JD, Won C, Kang CK, Kim GS. Inhibition of IAP's and activation of p53 leads to caspase-dependent apoptosis in gastric cancer cells treated with Scutellarein. Oncotarget. 2017 Dec 11;9(5):5993-6006. doi: 10.18632/oncotarget.23202. PMID: 29464049; PMCID: PMC5814189.

Li Y, Wang J, Zhong S, Li J, Du W. Scutellarein inhibits the development of colon cancer via CDC4-mediated RAGE ubiquitination. Int J Mol Med. 2020 Apr;45(4):1059-1072. doi: 10.3892/ijmm.2020.4496. Epub 2020 Feb 10. PMID: 32124957; PMCID: PMC7053863.

**Selenium-** is an essential mineral that has been studied to be able to prevent up to 25 percent of all cancers. It is found most abundantly in: brazil nuts, garlic, broccoli, and selenized yeast. It increases natural killer cells and macrophages, reduces angiogenesis, binds heavy metals, and activates glutathione. The areas in the US with the highest selenium in the soil have the lowest incidence of all cancers. There is a theory that those with cancer don't absorb selenium well, and thus may need higher doses to bring the blood levels up to normal. Glutathione peroxidase, the body's main internal antioxidant, requires selenium to function. About 400 mcg is the daily dose, but cancer patients may need higher levels. 4-6 brazil nuts per day is a great whole food dosage.

Vinceti M, Filippini T, Cilloni S, Crespi CM. The Epidemiology of Selenium and Human Cancer. Adv Cancer Res. 2017;136:1-48. doi: 10.1016/bs.acr.2017.07.001. Epub 2017 Aug 12. PMID: 29054414.

Rua RM, Nogales F, Carreras O, Ojeda ML. Selenium, selenoproteins and cancer of the thyroid. J Trace Elem Med Biol. 2023 Mar;76:127115. doi: 10.1016/j.jtemb.2022.127115. Epub 2022 Dec 5. PMID: 36481604.

Murdolo G, Bartolini D, Tortoioli C, Piroddi M, Torquato P, Galli F. Selenium and Cancer Stem Cells. Adv Cancer Res. 2017;136:235-257. doi: 10.1016/bs.acr.2017.07.006. Epub 2017 Oct 12. PMID: 29054420.

-T-

**Tangeritin-** is a flavonoid found in citrus fruits like tangerines and oranges, and has been found to have anti-cancer properties. In laboratory studies, tangeretin has been shown to inhibit the growth and spread of cancer cells in various types of cancer, including breast, leukemia, and prostate cancer. It works by inducing cell cycle arrest and apoptosis, or programmed cell death, in cancer cells. Tangeretin has also been found to have anti-inflammatory effects and can inhibit the formation of blood vessels that supply nutrients to cancer cells.

Raza W, Luqman S, Meena A. Prospects of tangeretin as a modulator of cancer targets/pathways. Pharmacol Res. 2020 Nov;161:105202. doi: 10.1016/j.phrs.2020.105202. Epub 2020 Sep 15. PMID: 32942013.

Gul HF, Ilhan N, Ilhan N, Ozercan IH, Kuloglu T. The combined effect of pomegranate extract and tangeretin on the DMBA-induced breast cancer model. J Nutr Biochem. 2021 Mar;89:108566. doi: 10.1016/j.jnutbio.2020.108566. Epub 2020 Dec 14. PMID: 33326843.

Dey DK, Chang SN, Vadlamudi Y, Park JG, Kang SC. Synergistic therapy with tangeretin and 5-fluorouracil accelerates the ROS/JNK mediated apoptotic pathway in human colorectal cancer cell. Food Chem Toxicol. 2020 Sep;143:111529. doi: 10.1016/j.fct.2020.111529. Epub 2020 Jun 30. PMID: 32619557.

**Theanine-** is a natural amino acid compound that is found mainly in green tea leaves and has been shown to have several health benefits. Recent studies have suggested that Theanine may have potential in the treatment and prevention of cancer due to its antioxidant and anti-inflammatory properties. Theanine has been shown to inhibit the growth and migration of cancer cells, including breast, lung, and colon cancer cells. It has also been shown to enhance the effectiveness of chemotherapy drugs while reducing their side effects. As a great bonus, it helps to reduce anxiety and increase mental focus.

Shojaei-Zarghani S, Rafraf M, Yari-Khosroushahi A. Theanine and cancer: A systematic review of the literature. Phytother Res. 2021 Sep;35(9):4782-4794. doi: 10.1002/ptr.7110. Epub 2021 Apr 23. PMID: 33891786.

Shojaei-Zarghani S, Yari Khosroushahi A, Rafraf M. Oncopreventive effects of theanine and theobromine on dimethylhydrazine-induced colon cancer model. Biomed Pharmacother. 2021 Feb;134:111140. doi: 10.1016/j.biopha.2020.111140. Epub 2020 Dec 24. PMID: 33360052.

Fan X, Zhou J, Bi X, Liang J, Lu S, Yan X, Luo L, Yin Z. L-theanine suppresses the metastasis of prostate cancer by downregulating MMP9 and Snail. J Nutr Biochem. 2021 Mar;89:108556. doi: 10.1016/j.jnutbio.2020.108556. Epub 2020 Nov 26. PMID: 33249185.

**Thymosin Alpha-1 (Tα1)-** is a synthetic version of a naturally occurring peptide hormone and has been studied for its role in cancer treatment and prevention. It is known to have immune-modulating effects that may help boost the immune system's ability to fight cancer. Several studies have shown that Tα1 may improve the efficacy of chemotherapy and radiation therapy in cancer patients. In addition, Tα1 has been found to have anti-inflammatory properties that could help reduce inflammation-associated cancer risk.

Wei Y, Zhang Y, Li P, Yan C, Wang L. Thymosin α-1 in cancer therapy: Immunoregulation and potential applications. Int Immunopharmacol. 2023 Apr;117:109744. doi: 10.1016/j.intimp.2023.109744. Epub 2023 Feb 20. PMID: 36812669.

Garaci E, Pica F, Sinibaldi-Vallebona P, Pierimarchi P, Mastino A, Matteucci C, Rasi G. Thymosin alpha(1) in combination with cytokines and chemotherapy for the treatment of cancer. Int Immunopharmacol. 2003 Aug;3(8):1145-50. doi: 10.1016/S1567-5769(03)00053-5. PMID: 12860169.

Wei YT, Wang XR, Yan C, Huang F, Zhang Y, Liu X, Wen ZF, Sun XT, Zhang Y, Chen YQ, Gao R, Pan N, Wang LX. Thymosin α-1 Reverses M2 Polarization of Tumor-Associated Macrophages during Efferocytosis. Cancer Res. 2022 May 16;82(10):1991-2002. doi: 10.1158/0008-5472.CAN-21-4260. PMID: 35364609.

**Thyroid hormone-** Balanced thyroid hormones play an important role in regulating various physiological functions, including cell growth, differentiation, and metabolism. Studies have shown that low levels of thyroid hormone are associated with an increased risk of developing certain types of cancer, such as breast and thyroid cancer. On the other hand, too-high levels of thyroid hormone have been linked to an increased risk of liver and colon cancer. Some research has also explored the potential use of thyroid hormone as an adjuvant therapy for cancer treatment. Overall, maintaining optimal levels of thyroid hormone through regular monitoring and treatment may help reduce the risk of certain types of cancer. As a general guideline, TSH should be between 1-2, and free T3 and free T4 levels within normal limits. Ask your doctor about ordering these tests.

Gauthier BR, Sola-García A, Cáliz-Molina MÁ, Lorenzo PI, Cobo-Vuilleumier N, Capilla-González V, Martin-Montalvo A. Thyroid hormones in diabetes, cancer, and aging. Aging Cell. 2020 Nov;19(11):e13260. doi: 10.1111/acel.13260. Epub 2020 Oct 13. PMID: 33048427; PMCID: PMC7681062.

Liu YC, Yeh CT, Lin KH. Molecular Functions of Thyroid Hormone Signaling in Regulation of Cancer Progression and Anti-Apoptosis. Int J Mol Sci. 2019 Oct 9;20(20):4986. doi: 10.3390/ijms20204986. Erratum in: Int J Mol Sci. 2020 Apr 30;21(9): PMID: 31600974; PMCID: PMC6834155.

Lin HY, Chin YT, Yang YC, Lai HY, Wang-Peng J, Liu LF, Tang HY, Davis PJ. Thyroid Hormone, Cancer, and Apoptosis. Compr Physiol. 2016 Jun 13;6(3):1221-37. doi: 10.1002/cphy.c150035. PMID: 27347891.

-U-

**Urea**- is a very affordable and non-toxic molecule. Orally it can be used for liver cancer and lung metastasis. Because of the way it is processed by the liver, oral supplementation does not help other areas of cancer, so it must be injected into the local tumor area. Clinically it has been shown to work synergistically with creatine supplements. This is the same creatine supplement that is often used for bodybuilding. Urea can be injected directly around the tumor and this can disrupt the glycoprotein layer and structured water around a tumor and prevent cancer cells from adhering together and growing properly. Topically, it can be used on skin cancers. Compounding pharmacies may be able to create a custom topical skin salve with urea for skin cancers.

Gandhi GM, Anasuya SR, Kawathekar P, Bhaskarmall, Krishnamurthy KR. Urea in the management of advanced malignancies (preliminary report). J Surg Oncol. 1977;9(2):139-46. doi: 10.1002/jso.2930090207. PMID: 266635.

Danopoulos ED, Chilaris GA, Danopoulou IE, Liaricos SB. Urea in the treatment of epibulbar malignancies. Br J Ophthalmol. 1975 May;59(5):282-7. doi: 10.1136/bjo.59.5.282. PMID: 1138858; PMCID: PMC1042617.

-V-

**Vitamin-D3**- has been linked to cancer prevention due to its ability to regulate cell growth, differentiation, and apoptosis. Studies suggest that vitamin D deficiency is associated with an increased risk of developing various types of cancer, including breast, prostate, and colorectal cancer. Additionally, research has shown that vitamin D supplementation may reduce the risk of cancer recurrence and improve cancer survival rates.
It can help with all cancers, but is critical for bone pain or bone metastasis, and for pain and fatigue in advanced cancer. Work with your doctor to get your levels between 40-60 (ng/mL) with blood testing.

Chirumbolo S. Vitamin D3 in cancer prevention and therapy: the nutritional issue. Horm Mol Biol Clin Investig. 2015 Sep;23(3):71-8. doi: 10.1515/hmbci-2015-0011. PMID: 26057218.

Carlberg C, Muñoz A. An update on vitamin D signaling and cancer. Semin Cancer Biol. 2022 Feb;79:217-230. doi: 10.1016/j.semcancer.2020.05.018. Epub 2020 May 30. PMID: 32485310.

Feldman D, Krishnan AV, Swami S, Giovannucci E, Feldman BJ. The role of vitamin D in reducing cancer risk and progression. Nat Rev Cancer. 2014 May;14(5):342-57. doi: 10.1038/nrc3691. Epub 2014 Apr 4. PMID: 24705652.

**Vitamin-C (IV-C)**- high-dose IV vitamin C has been studied for its use in cancer treatment and prevention. It is thought to work by producing hydrogen peroxide in cancer cells, which can lead to cell death. Additionally, vitamin C may help enhance the immune system's ability to fight cancer cells. Several clinical trials have been conducted to investigate the use of high-dose IV vitamin C alongside chemotherapy or radiation therapy in cancer treatment. In studies, patients had better life quality, lived longer, and had less nausea, fatigue, depression, and sleep disorders with concurrent IV-C therapy.

Klimant E, Wright H, Rubin D, Seely D, Markman M. Intravenous vitamin C in the supportive care of cancer patients: a review and rational approach. Curr Oncol. 2018 Apr;25(2):139-148. doi: 10.3747/co.25.3790. Epub 2018 Apr 30. PMID: 29719430; PMCID: PMC5927785.

Fritz H, Flower G, Weeks L, Cooley K, Callachan M, McGowan J, Skidmore B, Kirchner L, Seely D. Intravenous Vitamin C and Cancer: A Systematic Review. Integr Cancer Ther. 2014 Jul;13(4):280-300. doi: 10.1177/1534735414534463. Epub 2014 May 26. PMID: 24867961.

Magrì A, Germano G, Lorenzato A, Lamba S, Chilà R, Montone M, Amodio V, Ceruti T, Sassi F, Arena S, Abrignani S, D'Incalci M, Zucchetti M, Di Nicolantonio F, Bardelli A. High-dose vitamin C enhances cancer immunotherapy. Sci Transl Med. 2020 Feb 26;12(532):eaay8707. doi: 10.1126/scitranslmed.aay8707. PMID: 32102933.

**Vitamin K2**- plays a critical role in blood clotting and bone health. Recent studies suggest that vitamin K2 may also have anti-cancer properties. K2 works by inhibiting cancer cell growth and inducing cancer cell death. Some researchers have proposed that IV vitamin K2 may be a useful adjunct therapy for cancer treatment especially when combined with vitamin C.

Duan F, Mei C, Yang L, Zheng J, Lu H, Xia Y, Hsu S, Liang H, Hong L. Vitamin K2 promotes PI3K/AKT/HIF-1α-mediated glycolysis that leads to AMPK-dependent autophagic cell death in bladder cancer cells. Sci Rep. 2020 May 7;10(1):7714. doi: 10.1038/s41598-020-64880-x. PMID: 32382009; PMCID: PMC7206016.

Duan F, Yu Y, Guan R, Xu Z, Liang H, Hong L. Vitamin K2 Induces Mitochondria-Related Apoptosis in Human Bladder Cancer Cells via ROS and JNK/p38 MAPK Signal Pathways. PLoS One. 2016 Aug 29;11(8):e0161886. doi: 10.1371/journal.pone.0161886. PMID: 27570977; PMCID: PMC5003392.

-Z-

**Zinc-** is an essential mineral that plays a vital role in the immune system and has been shown to have anti-cancer properties. Studies have shown that zinc deficiency is common in cancer patients, and replenishing zinc levels can enhance the immune system and improve outcomes. Intravenous zinc therapy has been used in cancer patients as an adjunct to conventional therapies to improve their efficacy and reduce side effects. Zinc has also been shown to inhibit tumor growth and metastasis by inducing cell death and preventing cancer cell proliferation. Zinc is in a see-saw relationship with copper, so supplementing with extra zinc can help to drive down copper which is good because tumors can use extra copper to form new blood vessels in the angiogenesis process.

Skrajnowska D, Bobrowska-Korczak B. Role of Zinc in Immune System and Anti-Cancer Defense Mechanisms. Nutrients. 2019 Sep 22;11(10):2273. doi: 10.3390/nu11102273. PMID: 31546724; PMCID: PMC6835436.

To PK, Do MH, Cho JH, Jung C. Growth Modulatory Role of Zinc in Prostate Cancer and Application to Cancer Therapeutics. Int J Mol Sci. 2020 Apr 23;21(8):2991. doi: 10.3390/ijms21082991. PMID: 32340289; PMCID: PMC7216164.

Ho E, Song Y. Zinc and prostatic cancer. Curr Opin Clin Nutr Metab Care. 2009 Nov;12(6):640-5. doi: 10.1097/MCO.0b013e32833106ee. PMID: 19684515; PMCID: PMC4142760.

**2-Methoxyestradiol-** this is a methylated metabolite of estrogen that has been studied for its anticancer effects. It was approved as the drug Panzem, but this medication is taken orally and this creates unwanted metabolites when it passes through the liver. So this natural hormone can be more safely taken as a transdermal cream ordered through a compounding pharmacy.

Solum EJ, Akselsen ØW, Vik A, Hansen TV. Synthesis and Pharmacological Effects of the Anti-Cancer Agent 2-Methoxyestradiol. Curr Pharm Des. 2015;21(38):5453-66. doi: 10.2174/1381612821666151002112511. PMID: 26429718.

Gorska M, Kuban-Jankowska A, Slawek J, Wozniak M. New Insight into 2-Methoxyestradiol- a Possible Physiological Link between Neurodegeneration and Cancer Cell Death. Curr Med Chem. 2016;23(15):1513-27. doi: 10.2174/0929867323666160316123443. PMID: 26980569.

Varisli L. Decreased Expression of HN1 Sensitizes Prostate Cancer Cells to Apoptosis Induced by Docetaxel and 2-Methoxyestradiol. Ann Clin Lab Sci. 2022 Mar;52(2):196-201. PMID: 35414498.

## Chapter 9 Action Steps

Write in your journal or notebook:

- What are the supplements mentioned in this section that you may already have in your home?

- Which supplements have you already heard of, or seen at a health-food store?

- Which supplements have you never heard of that seem useful for your situation?

- Which supplements would you like to order now?

- Which supplements would you like to research more in depth?

# Chapter 10

## Molecular Pathway: Part 4- Mushrooms & Essential Oils

"Consuming mushrooms regularly has been associated with decreased risk of breast, stomach, and colorectal cancers."

-Dr Joel Fuhrman

### Medicinal Mushrooms

**Chaga (Inonotus obliquus)-** Chaga grows on birch trees and converts betulin to betulinic acid that has known anti-cancer effects. These fungi slow tumor growth, stimulate the immune system, slow metastasis, and kill cancer cells.

Lee MG, Kwon YS, Nam KS, Kim SY, Hwang IH, Kim S, Jang H. Chaga mushroom extract induces autophagy via the AMPK-mTOR signaling pathway in breast cancer cells. J Ethnopharmacol. 2021 Jun 28;274:114081. doi: 10.1016/j.jep.2021.114081. Epub 2021 Mar 30. PMID: 33798660.

Lee MG, Kwon YS, Nam KS, Kim SY, Hwang IH, Kim S, Jang H. Chaga mushroom extract induces autophagy via the AMPK-mTOR signaling pathway in breast cancer cells. J Ethnopharmacol. 2021 Jun 28;274:114081. doi: 10.1016/j.jep.2021.114081. Epub 2021 Mar 30. PMID: 33798660.

Nakajima Y, Nishida H, Matsugo S, Konishi T. Cancer cell cytotoxicity of extracts and small phenolic compounds from Chaga [Inonotus obliquus (persoon) Pilat]. J Med Food. 2009 Jun;12(3):501-7. doi: 10.1089/jmf.2008.1149. PMID: 19627197.

**Cordyceps (Cordyceps militaris)-** CS4 is an effective well-studied variety. It contains polysaccharides, nucleosides, and other bioactive components that show antioxidant and anti-inflammatory properties. These effects help in reducing oxidative stress and chronic inflammation, factors associated with cancer development. Studies have indicated that Cordyceps mushrooms possess anti-tumor effects by inhibiting cancer cell proliferation and promoting apoptosis in certain cancer types. It can also increase energy, lung capacity, and stamina to better endure the cancer treatment process.

Chen YY, Chen CH, Lin WC, Tung CW, Chen YC, Yang SH, Huang BM, Chen RJ. The Role of Autophagy in Anti-Cancer and Health Promoting Effects of Cordycepin. Molecules. 2021 Aug 16;26(16):4954. doi: 10.3390/molecules26164954. PMID: 34443541; PMCID: PMC8400201.

Quan X, Kwak BS, Lee JY, Park JH, Lee A, Kim TH, Park S. *Cordyceps militaris* Induces Immunogenic Cell Death and Enhances Antitumor Immunogenic Response in Breast Cancer. Evid Based Complement Alternat Med. 2020 Sep 3;2020:9053274. doi: 10.1155/2020/9053274. PMID: 32963576; PMCID: PMC7486645.

**Lion's Mane (Hericium erinaceus)**- These mushrooms slow tumor growth, stimulate the immune system, slow metastasis, and kill cancer cells. In addition, they stimulate nerve growth factor (NGF) in the brain and can help with memory, "chemo brain", and nerve repair in peripheral neuropathies.

Li W, Zhou W, Kim EJ, Shim SH, Kang HK, Kim YH. Isolation and identification of aromatic compounds in Lion's Mane Mushroom and their anticancer activities. Food Chem. 2015 Mar 1;170:336-42. doi: 10.1016/j.foodchem.2014.08.078. Epub 2014 Aug 23. PMID: 25306354.

Kim SP, Nam SH, Friedman M. Hericium erinaceus (Lion's Mane) mushroom extracts inhibit metastasis of cancer cells to the lung in CT-26 colon cancer-tansplanted mice. J Agric Food Chem. 2013 May 22;61(20):4898-904. doi: 10.1021/jf400916c. Epub 2013 May 13. Erratum in: J Agric Food Chem. 2013 Jun 5;61(22):5411. Erratum in: J Agric Food Chem. 2014 Jan 15;62(2):528. PMID: 23668749.

**Maitake (Grifola frondosa)**- These mushrooms are native to Japan and have been used as an adjunctive cancer treatment for many decades. They are known to help combat HIV, high blood pressure, diabetes, obesity, hepatitis, and cancer. The "D-fraction" is the most famous and well-studied constituent. It has synergistic effects with many chemotherapy drugs and radiation therapy.

Roldan-Deamicis A, Alonso E, Brie B, Braico DA, Balogh GA. Maitake Pro4X has anti-cancer activity and prevents oncogenesis in BALBc mice. Cancer Med. 2016 Sep;5(9):2427-41. doi: 10.1002/cam4.744. Epub 2016 Jul 11. PMID: 27401257; PMCID: PMC5055164.

Alonso EN, Ferronato MJ, Fermento ME, Gandini NA, Romero AL, Guevara JA, Facchinetti MM, Curino AC. Antitumoral and antimetastatic activity of Maitake D-Fraction in triple-negative breast cancer cells. Oncotarget. 2018 May 4;9(34):23396-23412. doi: 10.18632/oncotarget.25174. PMID: 29805742; PMCID: PMC5955106.

Wong JH, Ng TB, Chan HHL, Liu Q, Man GCW, Zhang CZ, Guan S, Ng CCW, Fang EF, Wang H, Liu F, Ye X, Rolka K, Naude R, Zhao S, Sha O, Li C, Xia L. Mushroom extracts and compounds with suppressive action on breast cancer: evidence from studies using cultured cancer cells, tumor-bearing animals, and clinical trials. Appl Microbiol Biotechnol. 2020 Jun;104(11):4675-4703. doi: 10.1007/s00253-020-10476-4. Epub 2020 Apr 9. PMID: 32274562.

**Reishi (Ganoderma lucidum)**- Is one of the most powerful mushrooms for the immune system. It supports the immune system to fight cancer better. It has even been studied to reverse chemotherapy resistance in cancer cells. And has synergistic effects when used along with chemo and radiation.

Unlu A, Nayir E, Kirca O, Ozdogan M. Ganoderma Lucidum (Reishi Mushroom) and cancer. J BUON. 2016 Jul-Aug;21(4):792-798. PMID: 27685898.

Jin X, Ruiz Beguerie J, Sze DM, Chan GC. Ganoderma lucidum (Reishi mushroom) for cancer treatment. Cochrane Database Syst Rev. 2016 Apr 5;4(4):CD007731. doi: 10.1002/14651858.CD007731.pub3. PMID: 27045603; PMCID: PMC6353236.

Cizmarikova M. The Efficacy and Toxicity of Using the Lingzhi or Reishi Medicinal Mushroom, Ganoderma lucidum (Agaricomycetes), and Its Products in Chemotherapy (Review). Int J Med Mushrooms. 2017;19(10):861-877. doi: 10.1615/IntJMedMushrooms.2017024537. PMID: 29256841.

**Shitake (Lentinus edodes)**- Is often used in Japanese cooking and has been studied for its cholesterol lowering and immune stimulating effects. It has the power to enhance the immune system, increase production of interferon, prevent chemical oncogenesis, and slow metastasis. Lentinan is the most studied molecule found in shiitake.

Ngai PH, Ng TB. Lentin, a novel and potent antifungal protein from shitake mushroom with inhibitory effects on activity of human immunodeficiency virus-1 reverse transcriptase and proliferation of leukemia cells. Life Sci. 2003 Nov 14;73(26):3363-74. doi: 10.1016/j.lfs.2003.06.023. PMID: 14572878.

Balakrishnan B, Liang Q, Fenix K, Tamang B, Hauben E, Ma L, Zhang W. Combining the Anticancer and Immunomodulatory Effects of Astragalus and Shiitake as an Integrated Therapeutic Approach. Nutrients. 2021 Jul 27;13(8):2564. doi: 10.3390/nu13082564. PMID: 34444724; PMCID: PMC8401741.

Xu T, Beelman RB, Lambert JD. The cancer preventive effects of edible mushrooms. Anticancer Agents Med Chem. 2012 Dec;12(10):1255-63. doi: 10.2174/187152012803833017. PMID: 22583406.

**Turkey Tail (Coriolus versicolor)**- Contains fractions called PSK & PSC that have been studied and used in Japan and China for decades as part of their conventional cancer treatment. Hot water extracts are best. It supports the immune system to fight cancer better, and has synergistic effects when used along with chemo and radiation.

Lowenthal R, Taylor M, Gidden JA, Heflin B, Lay JO Jr, Avaritt N, Tackett AJ, Urbaniak A. The mycelium of the Trametes versicolor synn. Coriolus versicolor (Turkey tail mushroom) exhibit anti-melanoma activity in vitro. Biomed Pharmacother. 2023 May;161:114424. doi: 10.1016/j.biopha.2023.114424. Epub 2023 Feb 22. PMID: 36827712; PMCID: PMC10147383.

Habtemariam S. Trametes versicolor (Synn. Coriolus versicolor) Polysaccharides in Cancer Therapy: Targets and Efficacy. Biomedicines. 2020 May 25;8(5):135. doi: 10.3390/biomedicines8050135. PMID: 32466253; PMCID: PMC7277906.

Pilkington K, Wieland LS, Teng L, Jin XY, Storey D, Liu JP. Coriolus (Trametes) versicolor mushroom to reduce adverse effects from chemotherapy or radiotherapy in people with colorectal cancer. Cochrane Database Syst Rev. 2022 Nov 29;11(11):CD012053. doi: 10.1002/14651858.CD012053.pub2. PMID: 36445793; PMCID: PMC9707730.

**Poria (Poria cocos)**- This is an ancient Chinese mushroom that contains polysaccharide molecules that can enhance the effectiveness of radiation and chemotherapy, stimulate the immune system, and inhibit the growth of tumors.

Qin L, Huang D, Huang J, Qin F, Huang H. Integrated Analysis and Finding Reveal Anti-Liver Cancer Targets and Mechanisms of Pachyman (*Poria cocos* Polysaccharides). Front Pharmacol. 2021 Sep 17;12:742349. doi: 10.3389/fphar.2021.742349. PMID: 34603055; PMCID: PMC8484528.

Li X, He Y, Zeng P, Liu Y, Zhang M, Hao C, Wang H, Lv Z, Zhang L. Molecular basis for Poria cocos mushroom polysaccharide used as an antitumour drug in China. J Cell Mol Med. 2019 Jan;23(1):4-20. doi: 10.1111/jcmm.13564. Epub 2018 Nov 15. PMID: 30444050; PMCID: PMC6307810.

Wang H, Luo Y, Chu Z, Ni T, Ou S, Dai X, Zhang X, Liu Y. Poria Acid, Triterpenoids Extracted from *Poria cocos*, Inhibits the Invasion and Metastasis of Gastric Cancer Cells. Molecules. 2022 Jun 6;27(11):3629. doi: 10.3390/molecules27113629. PMID: 35684565; PMCID: PMC9182142.

**White Button Mushrooms (Agaricus bisporus)**- have been studied to suppress cancer growth in prostate, lung, and stomach cancers. Certain compounds found in Agaricus bisporus, such as polysaccharides and phenolic compounds, exhibit antioxidant and immunomodulatory effects. Studies have demonstrated their ability to inhibit cancer cell growth, induce apoptosis, and potentially hinder tumor development.

Ankita Bhosale, Rashmi Trivedi, Tarun Kumar Upadhyay, Dhruvi Gurjar, Faranak Aghaz, Fahad Khan, Pratibha Pandey, Zeyaullah M, Alam MS, Al-Najjar MAA, Samra Siddiqui. Investigation on Antimicrobial, Antioxidant, and Anti-cancerous activity of Agaricus bisporus derived β-Glucan particles against cervical cancer cell line. Cell Mol Biol (Noisy-le-grand). 2022 Sep 30;68(9):150-159. doi: 10.14715/cmb/2022.68.9.24. PMID: 36905259.

Zhang N, Liu Y, Tang FY, Yang LY, Wang JH. Structural characterization and in vitro anti-colon cancer activity of a homogeneous polysaccharide from Agaricus bisporus. Int J Biol Macromol. 2023 Aug 18;251:126410. doi: 10.1016/j.ijbiomac.2023.126410. Epub ahead of print. PMID: 37598827.

Wang X, Ha D, Mori H, Chen S. White button mushroom (Agaricus bisporus) disrupts androgen receptor signaling in human prostate cancer cells and patient-derived xenograft. J Nutr Biochem. 2021 Mar;89:108580. doi: 10.1016/j.jnutbio.2020.108580. Epub 2020 Dec 31. PMID: 33388344; PMCID: PMC8542389.

## Essential Oils

Essential oils are powerfully concentrated plant medicines. Their molecules are so small that they easily evaporate into the air which is how they create the fragrances of different leaves, fruits, flowers, and bark of plants. These tiny molecules are also called terpenes. When studied individually most of these terpenes have shown anti-cancer effects and when combined in essential oil complexes they most likely have even more powerful synergistic anti-cancer properties. Because they're so concentrated, caution needs to be exercised in their use. All oils can be used in a diffuser as aromatherapy to breathe in and add healing molecules to the air of your home or car. All essential oils can be used topically to be absorbed through the skin, but some oils are better used when diluted in a carrier oil such as olive, coconut, or sweet almond oils, because they can cause burning or skin irritation if used straight. Oils that are more intense and require dilution before topical application include: oregano, thyme, cinnamon, clove, lemongrass, and peppermint. If you are using any essential oil for the first time, do a tiny drop test on your wrist first to make sure you don't have any sensitivities or allergic reactions. Citrus oils such as lemon, lime, orange, bergamot, and grapefruit can cause photosensitivity making your skin burn more easily when you go out into the sun. So use caution when going outside after using these oils. Most essential oils should not be used orally unless you know the company produces truly therapeutic grade oils. If you do decide to ingest essential oils, please do so under the direction of a skilled herbalist, aromatherapist, or naturopathic doctor, and only use reputable brands such as Plant Therapy, Edens Garden, and doTERRA, that are labeled therapeutic grade.

**Frankincense-** contains molecules such as: alpha-pinene, Limonene, alpha-Thujene, and beta-Pinene. Studies have suggested that these components possess anti-inflammatory, antioxidant, and anti-proliferative effects, which play a role in combating cancer cells. Research indicates that frankincense oil may interfere with cancer cell growth, induce apoptosis in various types of cancer cells, and inhibit angiogenesis.

Ren P, Ren X, Cheng L, Xu L. Frankincense, pine needle and geranium essential oils suppress tumor progression through the regulation of the AMPK/mTOR pathway in breast cancer. Oncol Rep. 2018 Jan;39(1):129-137. doi: 10.3892/or.2017.6067. Epub 2017 Nov 1. PMID: 29115548; PMCID: PMC5783593.

Reis D, Jones TT. Frankincense Essential Oil as a Supportive Therapy for Cancer-Related Fatigue: A Case Study. Holist Nurs Pract. 2018 May/Jun;32(3):140-142. doi: 10.1097/HNP.0000000000000261. PMID: 29642127.

Reis D, Throne T, Keller J, Koffel C, Chen T, Young-McCaughan S. Cancer-Related Fatigue: A Pilot Study Evaluating the Effect of Frankincense Essential Oil in Patients With Cancer Receiving Chemotherapy. Cancer Nurs. 2023 May-Jun 01;46(3):207-216. doi: 10.1097/NCC.0000000000001080. Epub 2022 Mar 3. PMID: 35245227.

**Eucalyptus**- contains 1,8-cineole, alpha-pinene, d-limonene and p-cymene, many of which have been studied for their anticancer effects. It has been studied to have cytotoxic effects in lung, colon, and liver cancers.

Khazraei H, Shamsdin SA, Zamani M. In Vitro Cytotoxicity and Apoptotic Assay of Eucalyptus globulus Essential Oil in Colon and Liver Cancer Cell Lines. J Gastrointest Cancer. 2022 Jun;53(2):363-369. doi: 10.1007/s12029-021-00601-5. Epub 2021 Mar 3. PMID: 33660226.

Anju, Kumar A, Yadav P, Navik U, Jaitak V. Chemical composition, *in vitro* and *in silico* evaluation of essential oil from *Eucalyptus tereticornis* leaves for lung cancer. Nat Prod Res. 2023 May;37(10):1656-1661. doi: 10.1080/14786419.2022.2107642. Epub 2022 Aug 8. PMID: 35938316.

**Peppermint**- Most of the research on peppermint oil has been on reducing the side effects of chemotherapy in helping with nausea, vomiting, and improving sleep quality. However, some preliminary research has shown direct cytotoxic and anti-tumor effects of peppermint oil

Hamzeh S, Safari-Faramani R, Khatony A. Effects of Aromatherapy with Lavender and Peppermint Essential Oils on the Sleep Quality of Cancer Patients: A Randomized Controlled Trial. Evid Based Complement Alternat Med. 2020 Mar 25;2020:7480204. doi: 10.1155/2020/7480204. PMID: 32308715; PMCID: PMC7132346.

Efe Ertürk N, Taşcı S. The Effects of Peppermint Oil on Nausea, Vomiting and Retching in Cancer Patients Undergoing Chemotherapy: An Open Label Quasi-Randomized Controlled Pilot Study. Complement Ther Med. 2021 Jan;56:102587. doi: 10.1016/j.ctim.2020.102587. Epub 2020 Oct 9. PMID: 33197662.

Silva WMF, Bona NP, Pedra NS, Cunha KFD, Fiorentini AM, Stefanello FM, Zavareze ER, Dias ARG. Risk assessment of in vitro cytotoxicity, antioxidant and antimicrobial activities of Mentha piperita

L. essential oil. J Toxicol Environ Health A. 2022 Mar 19;85(6):230-242. doi: 10.1080/15287394.2021.1999875. Epub 2021 Nov 15. PMID: 34781835.

**Sandalwood-** α-santalol is the most-studied molecule without known toxic side-effects. It has shown some anticancer effects in melanoma, breast and prostate cancer. Its ability to slow cancer-cell growth, and induce apoptosis in cancer cells are its most reported anticancer mechanisms of action.

Dozmorov MG, Yang Q, Wu W, Wren J, Suhail MM, Woolley CL, Young DG, Fung KM, Lin HK. Differential effects of selective frankincense (Ru Xiang) essential oil versus non-selective sandalwood (Tan Xiang) essential oil on cultured bladder cancer cells: a microarray and bioinformatics study. Chin Med. 2014 Jul 2;9:18. doi: 10.1186/1749-8546-9-18. PMID: 25006348; PMCID: PMC4086286.

Schwarztrauber M, Edwards N, Hiryak J, Chandrasekaran R, Wild J, Bommareddy A. Antitumor and chemopreventive role of major phytochemicals against breast cancer development. Nat Prod Res. 2023 Aug 30:1-21. doi: 10.1080/14786419.2023.2251167. Epub ahead of print. PMID: 37646820.

Dave K, Alsharif FM, Islam S, Dwivedi C, Perumal O. Chemoprevention of Breast Cancer by Transdermal Delivery of α-Santalol through Breast Skin and Mammary Papilla (Nipple). Pharm Res. 2017 Sep;34(9):1897-1907. doi: 10.1007/s11095-017-2198-z. Epub 2017 Jun 6. PMID: 28589445.

**Lavender-** its most abundant terpene is called linalool, and it has proven anticancer properties. In addition, Lavender is famous for helping induce relaxation, reduce stress, and promote healthy sleep which is critical for all cancer patients.

Duluklu B, Çelik SŞ. Effects of lavender essential oil for colorectal cancer patients with permanent colostomy on elimination of odor, quality of life, and ostomy adjustment: A randomized controlled trial. Eur J Oncol Nurs. 2019 Oct;42:90-96. doi: 10.1016/j.ejon.2019.08.001. Epub 2019 Aug 2. PMID: 31476706.

Boukhatem MN, Sudha T, Darwish NHE, Chader H, Belkadi A, Rajabi M, Houche A, Benkebailli F, Oudjida F, Mousa SA. A New Eucalyptol-Rich Lavender (*Lavandula stoechas* L.) Essential Oil: Emerging Potential for Therapy against Inflammation and Cancer. Molecules. 2020 Aug 12;25(16):3671. doi: 10.3390/molecules25163671. PMID: 32806608; PMCID: PMC7463424.

Şahin F, Özkaraman A, Irmak Kaya Z. The effect of a combined treatment of foot soak and lavender oil inhalation therapy on the severity of insomnia of patients with cancer: Randomized interventional study. Explore (NY). 2023 May-Jun;19(3):426-433. doi: 10.1016/j.explore.2022.09.003. Epub 2022 Sep 29. PMID: 36270928.

Zhao Y, Cheng X, Wang G, Liao Y, Qing C. Linalool inhibits 22Rv1 prostate cancer cell proliferation and induces apoptosis. Oncol Lett. 2020 Dec;20(6):289. doi: 10.3892/ol.2020.12152. Epub 2020 Sep 24. PMID: 33029205; PMCID: PMC7530887.

**Arbor Vitae**- some of this plant's molecules include: thujone, limonene, and pinene. These have all been studied individually to show anti-cancer effects.

Pudełek M, Catapano J, Kochanowski P, Mrowiec K, Janik-Olchawa N, Czyż J, Ryszawy D. Therapeutic potential of monoterpene α-thujone, the main compound of Thuja occidentalis L. essential oil, against malignant glioblastoma multiforme cells in vitro. Fitoterapia. 2019 Apr;134:172-181. doi: 10.1016/j.fitote.2019.02.020. Epub 2019 Feb 27. PMID: 30825580.

Lee JY, Park H, Lim W, Song G. Therapeutic potential of α,β-thujone through metabolic reprogramming and caspase-dependent apoptosis in ovarian cancer cells. J Cell Physiol. 2021 Feb;236(2):1545-1558. doi: 10.1002/jcp.30086. Epub 2020 Sep 30. PMID: 33000501.

Torres A, Vargas Y, Uribe D, Carrasco C, Torres C, Rocha R, Oyarzún C, San Martín R, Quezada C. Pro-apoptotic and anti-angiogenic properties of the α /β-thujone fraction from Thuja occidentalis on glioblastoma cells. J Neurooncol. 2016 May;128(1):9-19. doi: 10.1007/s11060-016-2076-2. Epub 2016 Feb 22. PMID: 26900077.

**Rosemary**- Rosemary oil demonstrates some of the most powerful antioxidant properties of any of the essential oils. It has world-famous effects at improving memory and cognition, and also shows direct anti-cancer effects in lab studies.

Ngo SN, Williams DB, Head RJ. Rosemary and cancer prevention: preclinical perspectives. Crit Rev Food Sci Nutr. 2011 Dec;51(10):946-54. doi: 10.1080/10408398.2010.490883. PMID: 21955093.

Melušová M, Jantová S, Horváthová E. Carvacrol and rosemary oil at higher concentrations induce apoptosis in human hepatoma HepG2 cells. Interdiscip Toxicol. 2014 Dec;7(4):189-94. doi: 10.2478/intox-2014-0027. Epub 2015 Mar 4. PMID: 26109899; PMCID: PMC4436207.

**Lemongrass**- contains terpenes such as myrcene, citral, and limonene that have shown anticancer properties in many lab studies.

Mukarram M, Choudhary S, Khan MA, Poltronieri P, Khan MMA, Ali J, Kurjak D, Shahid M. Lemongrass Essential Oil Components with Antimicrobial and Anticancer Activities. Antioxidants (Basel). 2021 Dec 22;11(1):20. doi: 10.3390/antiox11010020. PMID: 35052524; PMCID: PMC8773226.

Viktorová J, Stupák M, Řehořová K, Dobiasová S, Hoang L, Hajšlová J, Thanh TV, Tri LV, Tuan NV, Ruml T. Lemon Grass Essential Oil Does not Modulate Cancer Cells Multidrug Resistance by Citral-Its Dominant and Strongly Antimicrobial Compound. Foods. 2020 May 5;9(5):585. doi: 10.3390/foods9050585. PMID: 32380674; PMCID: PMC7278871.

Maruoka T, Kitanaka A, Kubota Y, Yamaoka G, Kameda T, Imataki O, Dobashi H, Bandoh S, Kadowaki N, Tanaka T. Lemongrass essential oil and citral inhibit Src/Stat3 activity and suppress the proliferation/survival of small-cell lung cancer cells, alone or in combination with chemotherapeutic agents. Int J Oncol. 2018 May;52(5):1738-1748. doi: 10.3892/ijo.2018.4314. Epub 2018 Mar 13. PMID: 29568932.

**Clove-** is most famous for its help in relieving pain and toothaches, but it also shows great potential in anti-cancer therapies.

Abadi AVM, Karimi E, Oskoueian E, Mohammad GRKS, Shafaei N. Chemical investigation and screening of anti-cancer potential of *Syzygium aromaticum* L. bud (clove) essential oil nanoemulsion. 3 Biotech. 2022 Feb;12(2):49. doi: 10.1007/s13205-022-03117-2. Epub 2022 Jan 27. PMID: 35127304; PMCID: PMC8795257.

Nirmala MJ, Durai L, Gopakumar V, Nagarajan R. Anticancer and antibacterial effects of a clove bud essential oil-based nanoscale emulsion system. Int J Nanomedicine. 2019 Aug 12;14:6439-6450. doi: 10.2147/IJN.S211047. PMID: 31496696; PMCID: PMC6697666.

**Basil-** basil is one of the most studied essential oils for cancer. It contains myrcene, eucalyptol, linalool, and eugenol among many other molecules. It has been shown to induce apoptosis in several cancer cell lines.

Bader A, Abdalla AN, Obaid NA, Youssef L, Naffadi HM, Elzubier ME, Almaimani RA, Flamini G, Pieracci Y, El-Readi MZ. In Vitro Anticancer and Antibacterial Activities of the Essential Oil of Forsskal's Basil Growing in Extreme Environmental Conditions. Life (Basel). 2023 Feb 26;13(3):651. doi: 10.3390/life13030651. PMID: 36983807; PMCID: PMC10057570.

Kathirvel P, Ravi S. Chemical composition of the essential oil from basil (Ocimum basilicum Linn.) and its in vitro cytotoxicity against HeLa and HEp-2 human cancer cell lines and NIH 3T3 mouse embryonic fibroblasts. Nat Prod Res. 2012;26(12):1112-8. doi: 10.1080/14786419.2010.545357. Epub 2011 Sep 22. PMID: 21939371.

Torres RG, Casanova L, Carvalho J, Marcondes MC, Costa SS, Sola-Penna M, Zancan P. Ocimum basilicum but not Ocimum gratissimum present cytotoxic effects on human breast cancer cell line MCF-7, inducing apoptosis and triggering mTOR/Akt/p70S6K pathway. J Bioenerg Biomembr. 2018 Apr;50(2):93-105. doi: 10.1007/s10863-018-9750-3. Epub 2018 Mar 28. PMID: 29589262.

**Geranium-** has anti-cancer growth, antiangiogenic, and anti-inflammatory properties. It contains geraniol and citral among other terpenes.

Boukhatem MN, Sudha T, Darwish NHE, Nada HG, Mousa SA. Essence aromatique du Géranium Odorant (Pelargonium graveolens L'Hérit.) d'Algérie : exploration des propriétés antioxydante, anti-inflammatoire et anticancéreuse (anti-angiogénique et cytotoxique), in vitro et in ovo, vis-à-vis de différentes lignées cellulaires cancéreuses métastasiques [Rose-scented geranium essential oil from Algeria (Pelargonium graveolens L'Hérit.): Assessment of antioxidant, anti-inflammatory and anticancer properties against different metastatic cancer cell lines]. Ann Pharm Fr. 2022 May;80(3):383-396. French. doi: 10.1016/j.pharma.2021.07.002. Epub 2021 Jul 24. PMID: 34310905.

Ren P, Ren X, Cheng L, Xu L. Frankincense, pine needle and geranium essential oils suppress tumor progression through the regulation of the AMPK/mTOR pathway in breast cancer. Oncol Rep. 2018 Jan;39(1):129-137. doi: 10.3892/or.2017.6067. Epub 2017 Nov 1. PMID: 29115548; PMCID: PMC5783593.

**Clary sage-** is known to contain molecules such as sclareol, ferruginol, and salvipisone. These molecules have shown to be toxic to cancer cells in several lab studies.

Hayet E, Fatma B, Souhir I, Waheb FA, Abderaouf K, Mahjoub A, Maha M. Antibacterial and cytotoxic activity of the acetone extract of the flowers of Salvia sclarea and some natural products. Pak J Pharm Sci. 2007 Apr;20(2):146-8. PMID: 17416571.

Zhou J, Xie X, Tang H, Peng C, Peng F. The bioactivities of sclareol: A mini review. Front Pharmacol. 2022 Oct 3;13:1014105. doi: 10.3389/fphar.2022.1014105. PMID: 36263135; PMCID: PMC9574335.

Rózalski M, Kuźma L, Krajewska U, Wysokińska H. Cytotoxic and proapoptotic activity of diterpenoids from in vitro cultivated Salvia sclarea roots. Studies on the leukemia cell lines. Z Naturforsch C J Biosci. 2006 Jul-Aug;61(7-8):483-8. doi: 10.1515/znc-2006-7-804. PMID: 16989306.

**Lemon-** has limonene and citral as its most abundant terpenes, both of which have been studied to fight cancer. It can induce apoptosis and reduce angiogenesis.

Yousefian Rad E, Homayouni Tabrizi M, Ardalan P, Seyedi SMR, Yadamani S, Zamani-Esmati P, Haghani Sereshkeh N. *Citrus lemon* essential oil nanoemulsion (CLEO-NE), a safe cell-depended apoptosis inducer in human A549 lung cancer cells with anti-angiogenic activity. J Microencapsul. 2020 Aug;37(5):394-402. doi: 10.1080/02652048.2020.1767223. Epub 2020 May 19. PMID: 32400238.

Petretto GL, Vacca G, Addis R, Pintore G, Nieddu M, Piras F, Sogos V, Fancello F, Zara S, Rosa A. Waste *Citrus limon* Leaves as Source of Essential Oil Rich in Limonene and Citral: Chemical Characterization, Antimicrobial and Antioxidant Properties, and Effects on Cancer Cell Viability.

Antioxidants (Basel). 2023 Jun 8;12(6):1238. doi: 10.3390/antiox12061238. PMID: 37371968; PMCID: PMC10295007.

**Grapefruit-** contains the molecules limonene, α-pinene, and myrcene which have all demonstrated anticancer effects.

Deng W, Liu K, Cao S, Sun J, Zhong B, Chun J. Chemical Composition, Antimicrobial, Antioxidant, and Antiproliferative Properties of Grapefruit Essential Oil Prepared by Molecular Distillation. Molecules. 2020 Jan 5;25(1):217. doi: 10.3390/molecules25010217. PMID: 31948058; PMCID: PMC6982870.

Zhao Y, Chen R, Wang Y, Yang Y. α-Pinene Inhibits Human Prostate Cancer Growth in a Mouse Xenograft Model. Chemotherapy. 2018;63(1):1-7. doi: 10.1159/000479863. Epub 2017 Oct 26. PMID: 29069647.

**Lime-** has the terpenes limonene, cineole, pinene, and citral as well as others. Each has demonstrated anticancer effects in numerous lab studies.

Klauser AL, Hirschfeld M, Ritter A, Rücker G, Jäger M, Gundarova J, Weiss D, Juhasz-Böss I, Berner K, Erbes T, Asberger J. Anticarcinogenic Effects of Odorant Substances Citral, Citrathal R and Cyclovertal on Breast Cancer in vitro. Breast Cancer (Dove Med Press). 2021 Dec 8;13:659-673. doi: 10.2147/BCTT.S322619. PMID: 34916844; PMCID: PMC8668161.

Murata S, Shiragami R, Kosugi C, Tezuka T, Yamazaki M, Hirano A, Yoshimura Y, Suzuki M, Shuto K, Ohkohchi N, Koda K. Antitumor effect of 1, 8-cineole against colon cancer. Oncol Rep. 2013 Dec;30(6):2647-52. doi: 10.3892/or.2013.2763. Epub 2013 Oct 1. PMID: 24085263.

Hou J, Zhang Y, Zhu Y, Zhou B, Ren C, Liang S, Guo Y. α-Pinene Induces Apoptotic Cell Death via Caspase Activation in Human Ovarian Cancer Cells. Med Sci Monit. 2019 Sep 4;25:6631-6638. doi: 10.12659/MSM.916419. PMID: 31482864; PMCID: PMC6743669.

**Orange**- sweet orange oil was studied to be the highest source of the anticancer molecule limonene. One study showed the ability of orange oil to reduce angiogenesis, metastasis, and cancer-cell viability.

Liu K, Deng W, Hu W, Cao S, Zhong B, Chun J. Extraction of 'Gannanzao' Orange Peel Essential Oil by Response Surface Methodology and its Effect on Cancer Cell Proliferation and Migration. Molecules. 2019 Jan 30;24(3):499. doi: 10.3390/molecules24030499. PMID: 30704118; PMCID: PMC6384855.

Chidambara Murthy KN, Jayaprakasha GK, Patil BS. D-limonene rich volatile oil from blood oranges inhibits angiogenesis, metastasis and cell death in human colon cancer cells. Life Sci. 2012 Oct 5;91(11-12):429-439. doi: 10.1016/j.lfs.2012.08.016. Epub 2012 Aug 20. PMID: 22935404.

Yang C, Chen H, Chen H, Zhong B, Luo X, Chun J. Antioxidant and Anticancer Activities of Essential Oil from Gannan Navel Orange Peel. Molecules. 2017 Aug 22;22(8):1391. doi: 10.3390/molecules22081391. PMID: 28829378; PMCID: PMC6152265.

**Rose**- these famous flowers contain citronellol, geraniol, and nerol which have some demonstrated anticancer effects.

Rezaie-Tavirani M, Fayazfar S, Heydari-Keshel S, Rezaee MB, Zamanian-Azodi M, Rezaei-Tavirani M, Khodarahmi R. Effect of essential oil of Rosa Damascena on human colon cancer cell line SW742. Gastroenterol Hepatol Bed Bench. 2013 Winter;6(1):25-31. PMID: 24834241; PMCID: PMC4017490.

Yu WN, Lai YJ, Ma JW, Ho CT, Hung SW, Chen YH, Chen CT, Kao JY, Way TD. Citronellol Induces Necroptosis of Human Lung Cancer Cells via TNF-α Pathway and Reactive Oxygen Species Accumulation. In Vivo. 2019 Jul-Aug;33(4):1193-1201. doi: 10.21873/invivo.11590. PMID: 31280209; PMCID: PMC6689369.

Shokrzadeh M, Habibi E, Modanloo M. Cytotoxic and genotoxic studies of essential oil from Rosa damascene Mill., Kashan, Iran. Med Glas (Zenica). 2017 Aug 1;14(2):152-157. doi: 10.17392/901-17. PMID: 28644429.

**Thyme-** has medicinal molecules that include: thymol, carvacrol, linalool, and caryophyllene. These components have been shown to kill cancer cells.

Vassiliou E, Awoleye O, Davis A, Mishra S. Anti-Inflammatory and Antimicrobial Properties of Thyme Oil and Its Main Constituents. Int J Mol Sci. 2023 Apr 8;24(8):6936. doi: 10.3390/ijms24086936. PMID: 37108100; PMCID: PMC10138399.

Niksic H, Becic F, Koric E, Gusic I, Omeragic E, Muratovic S, Miladinovic B, Duric K. Cytotoxicity screening of Thymus vulgaris L. essential oil in brine shrimp nauplii and cancer cell lines. Sci Rep. 2021 Jun 23;11(1):13178. doi: 10.1038/s41598-021-92679-x. PMID: 34162964; PMCID: PMC8222331.

**Winter Savory & Summer Savory-** this unique kitchen herb contains carvacrol, pinene, myrcene, thymol, linalool, and caryophyllene. These have all been studied for their anticancer effects. They have some of the best results for the most cancer types out of the essential oils that have been studied so far.

Moreira SA, Silva S, Costa E, Pinto S, Sarmento B, Saraiva JA, Pintado M. Effect of High Hydrostatic Pressure Extraction on Biological Activities and Phenolics Composition of Winter Savory Leaf Extracts. Antioxidants (Basel). 2020 Sep 8;9(9):841. doi: 10.3390/antiox9090841. PMID: 32911721; PMCID: PMC7554779.

Butnariu M, Quispe C, Herrera-Bravo J, Helon P, Kukula-Koch W, López V, Les F, Vergara CV, Alarcón-Zapata P, Alarcón-Zapata B, Martorell M, Pentea M, Dragunescu AA, Samfira I, Yessimsiitova Z, Daştan SD, Castillo CMS, Roberts TH, Sharifi-Rad J, Koch W, Cho WC. The effects of thymoquinone on pancreatic cancer: Evidence from preclinical studies. Biomed Pharmacother. 2022 Sep;153:113364. doi: 10.1016/j.biopha.2022.113364. Epub 2022 Jul 8. PMID: 35810693.

Kundaković T, Stanojković T, Kolundzija B, Marković S, Sukilović B, Milenković M, Lakusić B. Cytotoxicity and antimicrobial activity of the essential oil from Satureja montana subsp. pisidica (Lamiceae). Nat Prod Commun. 2014 Apr;9(4):569-72. PMID: 24868886.

**Balsam Fir-** contains the active molecules α-pinene, β-pinene, β-phellandrene, and limonene. These constituents have been studied for their effects at reducing cancer pain, to synergize with certain chemo drugs, and stimulate the immune cells that kill cancer.

Pinheiro-Neto FR, Lopes EM, Acha BT, Gomes LDS, Dias WA, Reis Filho ACD, Leal BS, Rodrigues DCDN, Silva JDN, Dittz D, Ferreira PMP, Almeida FRC. α-Phellandrene exhibits antinociceptive and tumor-reducing effects in a mouse model of oncologic pain. Toxicol Appl Pharmacol. 2021 May 1;418:115497. doi: 10.1016/j.taap.2021.115497. Epub 2021 Mar 17. PMID: 33744277.

Lin JJ, Lu KW, Ma YS, Tang NY, Wu PP, Wu CC, Lu HF, Lin JG, Chung JG. Alpha-phellandrene, a natural active monoterpene, influences a murine WEHI-3 leukemia model in vivo by enhancing macrophague phagocytosis and natural killer cell activity. In Vivo. 2014 Jul-Aug;28(4):583-8. PMID: 24982226.

Zhang Z, Guo S, Liu X, Gao X. Synergistic antitumor effect of α-pinene and β-pinene with paclitaxel against non-small-cell lung carcinoma (NSCLC). Drug Res (Stuttg). 2015 Apr;65(4):214-8. doi: 10.1055/s-0034-1377025. Epub 2014 Sep 4. PMID: 25188609.

**Bergamot**- this relative of oranges is a symphony of healing molecules including: limonene, linalool, terpinene, and β-pinene. It has proven anti-inflammatory, antioxidant, and anticancer effects.

Celia C, Trapasso E, Locatelli M, Navarra M, Ventura CA, Wolfram J, Carafa M, Morittu VM, Britti D, Di Marzio L, Paolino D. Anticancer activity of liposomal bergamot essential oil (BEO) on human neuroblastoma cells. Colloids Surf B Biointerfaces. 2013 Dec 1;112:548-53. doi: 10.1016/j.colsurfb.2013.09.017. Epub 2013 Sep 17. PMID: 24099646.

Adorisio S, Muscari I, Fierabracci A, Thi Thuy T, Marchetti MC, Ayroldi E, Delfino DV. Biological effects of bergamot and its potential therapeutic use as an anti-inflammatory, antioxidant, and anticancer agent. Pharm Biol. 2023 Dec;61(1):639-646. doi: 10.1080/13880209.2023.2197010. PMID: 37067190; PMCID: PMC10114982.

**Pine**- contains terpineol, linalool, limonene, caryophyllene, and eugenol all of which have demonstrated anticancer effects.

Thalappil MA, Butturini E, Carcereri de Prati A, Bettin I, Antonini L, Sapienza FU, Garzoli S, Ragno R, Mariotto S. *Pinus mugo* Essential Oil Impairs STAT3 Activation through Oxidative Stress and Induces Apoptosis in Prostate Cancer Cells. Molecules. 2022 Jul 28;27(15):4834. doi: 10.3390/molecules27154834. PMID: 35956786; PMCID: PMC9369512.

Hoai NT, Duc HV, Thao do T, Orav A, Raal A. Selectivity of Pinus sylvestris extract and essential oil to estrogen-insensitive breast cancer cells Pinus sylvestris against cancer cells. Pharmacogn Mag. 2015 Oct;11(Suppl 2):S290-5. doi: 10.4103/0973-1296.166052. PMID: 26664017; PMCID: PMC4653339.

Zhang Y, Xin C, Qiu J, Wang Z. Essential Oil from *Pinus Koraiensis* Pinecones Inhibits Gastric Cancer Cells via the HIPPO/YAP Signaling Pathway. Molecules. 2019 Oct 25;24(21):3851. doi: 10.3390/molecules24213851. PMID: 31731517; PMCID: PMC6864528.

**Cypress**- has been shown to contain pinene, carene, limonene, and α-terpinolene. These anticancer molecules have been studied in dozens of scientific papers.

Aydin E, Türkez H, Taşdemir S. Anticancer and antioxidant properties of terpinolene in rat brain cells. Arh Hig Rada Toksikol. 2013 Sep;64(3):415-24. doi: 10.2478/10004-1254-64-2013-2365. PMID: 24084350.

Yoshida N, Takada T, Yamamura Y, Adachi I, Suzuki H, Kawakami J. Inhibitory effects of terpenoids on multidrug resistance-associated protein 2- and breast cancer resistance protein-mediated transport. Drug Metab Dispos. 2008 Jul;36(7):1206-11. doi: 10.1124/dmd.107.019513. Epub 2008 Apr 24. PMID: 18436619.

**Spearmint**- contains the medicinal components carvone, carveol, dihydrocarvone, dihydrocarveol. This mint family oil can prevent and treat breast as well as other cancers.

Tubtimsri S, Limmatvapirat C, Limsirichaikul S, Akkaramongkolporn P, Inoue Y, Limmatvapirat S. Fabrication and characterization of spearmint oil loaded nanoemulsions as cytotoxic agents against oral cancer cell. Asian J Pharm Sci. 2018 Sep;13(5):425-437. doi: 10.1016/j.ajps.2018.02.003. Epub 2018 Mar 16. PMID: 32104417; PMCID: PMC7032207.

Rasti F, Yousefpoor Y, Abdollahi A, Safari M, Roozitalab G, Osanloo M. Antioxidative, anticancer, and antibacterial activities of a nanogel containing Mentha spicata L. essential oil and electrospun nanofibers of polycaprolactone-hydroxypropyl methylcellulose. BMC Complement Med Ther. 2022 Oct 7;22(1):261. doi: 10.1186/s12906-022-03741-8. PMID: 36207726; PMCID: PMC9540714.

Crowell PL. Monoterpenes in breast cancer chemoprevention. Breast Cancer Res Treat. 1997 Nov-Dec;46(2-3):191-7. doi: 10.1023/a:1005939806591. PMID: 9478274.

## Essential Oil Affinities For Specific Cancers

**Bone**- frankincense, helichrysum, white fir, lemmon

**Brain**- frankincense, clove, myrrh, arborvitae,

**Breast**- rosemary, lavender, frankincense, arbor vitae, Clary sage, clove, basil, sandalwood, oregano, lemongrass, marjoram

**Cervical**- frankincense, geranium, white fir, Cypress, clove, lavender, lemon, rosemary

**Colon**- Lavender, geranium, frankincense, arborvitae, lemongrass

**Leukemia**- frankincense, lemongrass, rosemary, Clary sage, clove, lemon, sandalwood

**Liver**- frankincense, lemongrass, lavender, rosemary, geranium, clove, thyme

**Lung**- frankincense, lavender, Melissa, eucalyptus, thyme

**Lymphoma**- wild orange, frankincense, thyme, clove

**Ovarian**- geranium, Clary sage, frankincense, rosemary

**Pancreas**- frankincense, coriander, coriander, clove

**Prostate**- frankincense, arborvitae, oregano,

**Skin**- sandalwood, arbor vitae, frankincense, lemon, lime, orange, grapefruit, geranium,

**Throat**- frankincense, lavender, cinnamon, thyme

**Uterine**- geranium, frankincense, Clary sage, rosemary

## Chapter 10 Action Steps

Choose one medicinal mushroom or a mushroom formula to start taking this week.

Choose 3-5 essential oils to begin to use. Combine these oils with a carrier oil such as olive, coconut, or almond and use this blend for a full body massage on a regular basis. You can use the oils with scents that you enjoy the most in an aromatherapy diffuser throughout the day. This will add more medicinal molecules to the air that will get into your bloodstream through your nose, lungs, and skin.

# Chapter 11

## Molecular Pathway: Part 5-Lab Testing

"We see a day where people are screened with a simple blood draw for many cancers ... That dream is closer to reality than I think any of us fully appreciate."

- Kevin Conroy, president Exact Sciences

The world of Labs is constantly changing, and many labs and tests come and go as the research and business climate changes. This list is current as of the time of this writing in 2025, but I cannot guarantee that these labs will remain open or offer the same tests in coming years. Many of these are offered by mainstream medical labs like Quest Diagnostics and Labcorp, while others are offered only by the specific companies listed in the 2nd half of the chapter.

### Specific Lab Tests

Some of these you can order yourself, and others will require going through a licensed healthcare provider.

**Urine Heavy Metals**- This test can measure levels of lead, mercury cadmium, and other toxic metals that are excreted in your urine. High levels of these toxic elements can cause disease and malfunction in the body and contribute to the cancer process. If high levels are found, work with a professional trained in chelation therapy or Naturopathic detoxification to safely reduce levels of these metals.

**Urine Mold Toxins**- Mold toxicity is a common condition that many people are not aware that they have. You can have mold exposure from eating, touching, or breathing in mold spores. These molds then produce molecules called mycotoxins that are excreted in the urine and can be measured to assess your toxic load. The book *Toxic* by Dr Neil Nathan is a fantastic resource for this condition.

**Urine Toxic Chemicals**- This lab panel measures excreted levels of common cancer-causing chemicals such as benzene, phthalates, pesticides, herbicides, and other toxic molecules.

**Food Sensitivity Testing**- This can provide a snapshot of the foods that your immune system is currently reacting to. If the list is very large this means you most likely have problems with leaky gut, or intestinal permeability, of too many undigested proteins getting through the intestinal wall and causing the immune system to react as if the foods are foreign invaders. If you eliminate these reactive foods for at least 6 months it can give your immune system a chance to catch up and focus on the cancer process instead of fighting normal food molecules that have gotten into your bloodstream.

**Blood Micronutrient Testing**- Micronutrients are the microscopic: vitamins, minerals, and fatty acids needed for a healthy body. This test can pinpoint specific deficiencies in your system that can be filled with certain foods or supplements to make sure your individual nutritional needs are being met.

**Inflammation testing**- C-Reactive Protein (CRP), High-sensitivity C-Reactive Protein (HS-CRP), and Erythrocyte sedimentation Rate (ESR) are all blood tests that measure inflammation in the body. Elevated levels of inflammation are linked to higher risks of being diagnosed with cancer, and cancer is made worse by higher levels of inflammation as well. These tests can give a baseline inflammation level, and then you can assess the success of your anti-inflammatory diet and lifestyle choices with repeated testing.

**Albumin**- This is a protein found on the Complete Metabolic Panel (CMP) Test. It is made by the liver and is important for maintaining the body's fluid balance and transporting various substances, such as hormones and medications, throughout the body. In cancer, low levels of albumin, known as hypoalbuminemia, can be a common finding and may be associated with poor prognosis and reduced overall survival. Hypoalbuminemia can

occur due to various reasons, including malnutrition, inflammation, and liver dysfunction.

In cancer patients, it can also be a sign of advanced disease and poor response to treatment. Albumin levels may be used as a marker for assessing the nutritional status and overall health of cancer patients, and addressing albumin deficiencies through nutritional support or other interventions may help improve treatment outcomes.

**Insulin Like Growth Factor 1 (IGF1)-** This is a growth factor made in the body that influences levels of human growth hormone (HGH). It is found to be high in a number of cancers. Diet and lifestyle factors can influence your levels of IGF1, and therefore your levels of cancer risk. My understanding is that if you are healthy, IGF1 and growth hormone are supportive of health and help you build muscle, burn fat, and repair injuries, but if you are unhealthy or have cancer, then it is like adding Miracle Grow to the cancer cells, because its job is to help cells grow faster. So if you have cancer, you want your IGF1 levels to be on the lowest end of the normal range.

**Galectin-3** Is a protein made in the body, but is overexpressed when you have cancer. When it is high, modified citrus pectin supplements can bind and remove the excess Galectin-3 from the system, and reduce the cancer process.

**Tests For Blood Clotting-** Plasminogen Activator Inhibitor (PAI1), Fibrinogen, D-dimer- These tests all determine if there is an issue with too much clotting, or blood coagulability. The cancer process almost always creates a state of increased clotting in the blood, so these tests can determine the extent of this process and how much intervention is needed to correct it.

**Copper-** This is the metal copper that is needed by the body in small amounts for brain development, making energy, and in building new

connective tissues and blood vessels. As you have read about earlier, angiogenesis is the process of the body creating new blood vessels.

Tumors need copper to create new blood vessels to supply themselves with blood to maintain and grow. Thus lowering copper is a therapeutic target to help slow down the process of angiogenesis.

**Ceruloplasmin-** Is a protein that acts as a shuttle bus to store and carry copper to where it needs to go in the body. Because of the role of copper in angiogenesis that can support tumor growth, doctors like to see this value as low as possible without creating other symptoms.

**Zinc-** Zinc has many beneficial effects on the cancer process. First, zinc has a see-saw relationship with copper in the body, so if you supplement with zinc, copper will go down, which helps reduce the copper available for angiogenesis. Zinc is also an essential mineral for immune health, and supports apoptosis or programmed cancer cell death. So you want to have zinc levels at the high end of the normal range of testing.

**Lactate Dehydrogenase (LDH)-** LDH is an enzyme found in most cells in the body that is used to process lactate that forms a result of metabolizing glucose for fuel. Cancer cells use more glucose and make more lactate acid than normal cells, so this will be elevated in active cancers. This test is not specific to any certain type of cancer, and it is not specific to cancer in general since there are many diseases that can also raise LDH levels, however it can be a useful clue to monitor cancer treatment progress or recurrence.

**Fasting insulin-** This is the measurement of the hormone insulin that is released by the pancreas in response to consuming carbohydrates. Under 10 is the ideal for cancer patients. This is an indicator that you are keeping a healthy level of blood glucose and don't have any insulin resistance that can worsen the cancer process.

**Hemoglobin A1c-** This is the same marker that is used to monitor diabetes treatment. It's a measurement of your average blood glucose levels over the past 3 months or so. Under 5.5 is the ideal. Since cancer cells are so

dependent on blood glucose for fuel, you want this to be as low as you can to support your body's efforts to heal. If you have an A1c reading above 5.5, then decrease your intake of sugars, flours, and sweet fruits, and increase your intake of healthy fats (olives, avocados, nuts, coconut, etc) and fiber (vegetables, beans, lentils).

**High-Sensitivity Human Chorionic Gonadotropin-** (HS HCG) (blood or urine test)- This is the same protein that is detected in pregnancy tests. Men or non-pregnant women should not have any detectable levels of HCG in their blood or urine. Cancer cells revert back to a state similar to an embryo and therefore make this embryonic protein. This test can be used to assess for a cancer recurrence as well as monitor treatment progress. Navaro in the Philippines offers this urine test. Many labs in the US offer the quantitative blood test for HCG, which can be used for the same purposes.

**Phosphohexose Isomerase (PHI)** - is an enzyme that is an indicator of increased glycolysis (using up blood glucose) that is higher in cancer cells. This test is included in the American Metabolic Laboratories Cancer Profile described later.

**Pyruvate kinase-** is an enzyme in the body that comes in 2 forms, PKM1 and PKM2. Cancer cells express higher levels of the PKM2 form, so it can be used as a cancer marker to measure treatment success.

**NK Cell Activity Test-** Natural Killer or NK Cells are a powerful part of your immune system that target and kill cancer cells. These tests can assess how active your NK cells are so you can adjust therapy to influence your NK Cell function.

**Ki67-** If you have a biopsy taken, you can ask your doctor to run a KI-67 test that shows what percentage of cells are actively dividing. This is an indication of how active or aggressive your cancer currently is. Treatment can be modified to be more aggressive when this number is higher.

## Laboratories That Do Testing

**Galleri-** Is a company offering an innovative blood test for early detection of 50+ different types of cancer. Early detection usually leads to better clinical outcomes unless doctors jump into aggressive conventional treatment too quickly. This too early aggressive treatment can sometimes cause more harm than good in early cancers that may not have ever become dangerous. https://www.galleri.com/

**Weisenthal Cancer Group**- When a patient has an infection, it is common practice for a doctor to run a culture and sensitivity test. This means they take your blood or urine and grow the bacteria they find there in a lab, then they run tests on it to see which antibiotics will best kill your specific bacterial infection.

Chemosensitivity testing is the same principle, but with cancer cells. When you have a biopsy taken, part of it is overnight shipped to this lab and they run tests to see which chemotherapies and natural agents kill your actual cancer cells most effectively. This can be a lifesaving test, and more oncologists need to be informed about its availability and use. http://www.weisenthalcancer.com

**Research Genetics Cancer Center (RGCC)**- Has several advanced cancer profiles that can be run to obtain critical information about your specific cancer. They can test for circulating cancer cells which can provide an early diagnosis or monitor treatment. They also perform chemosensitivity testing to assess which chemotherapies and natural substances your specific cancer cells are most sensitive to. https://rgcc-international.com

**Precision Oncology**- Has several panels including the Oncotype dx panel that can help assess the likelihood of a recurrence of breast or colon cancer after initial treatment. https://precisiononcology.exactsciences.com

**Cologuard**- Is a stool test for both hidden blood and altered DNA that are usually found in colon cancer. There are risks that come with colonoscopies, so this is an alternative non-invasive screening test for colon cancer. https://www.cologuard.com/

**American Metabolic Laboratories**- Offers a Cancer Profile© that includes: **HCG** (human chorionic gonadotropin hormone) X2, **PHI** (phosphohexose isomerase), **GGTP** (gamma-glutamyl transpeptidase) enzyme, **CEA** (carcinoembryonic antigen), **TSH** (thyroid stimulating hormone), and **DHEA-S** (dehydroepiandrosterone sulfate), the adrenal "anti-stress, pro-immunity and longevity hormone".

This profile costs $719 and is one of the only labs in the U.S. that offers high-sensitivity HCG which is a protein made by almost all cancer cells. It also includes many other cancer markers that increase the odds of a proper diagnosis.

**Dutch Hormone Testing**- Offers a comprehensive urinary hormone panel that will be important for the treatment of any hormonally dependent cancers like breast, ovarian, and prostate.

## Chapter 11 Action Steps

Find a Naturopathic Doctor, Medical Doctor, or Nurse Practitioner who is willing to work with you in ordering the tests that you are interested in pursuing and that you can afford. There are many telemedicine options now that were not available just a few years ago. Ask your insurance provider which tests they will cover and which will be out of pocket.

## Resources

### Books:

**Toxic** -Dr Neil Nathan  (Reducing the burden of mold, lyme disease, and other mystery illness)

**The Survival Paradox** -Dr Issac Eliaz   (Explains the role of Galectin-3 in cancer and other diseases and the role of Modified Citrus Pectin in binding and excreting Galectin-3)

### Labs:

https://www.anylabtestnow.com/

https://www.cologuard.com/

https://americanmetaboliclaboratories.com/services/

https://precisiononcology.exactsciences.com/

https://rgcc-international.com

http://www.weisenthalcancer.com

https://www.galleri.com/

https://www.greatplainslaboratory.com/

https://www.cyrexlabs.com/

https://www.doctorsdata.com/

https://dutchtest.com/

# Chapter 12

## The Molecular Pathway: Part 6- The Molecules to Avoid

*"The war on cancer set out to find, treat, and cure a disease-but it has left untouched many of the things known to cause cancer, including tobacco, the workplace, radiation, and the global environment."*

-Devra Davis author of, *The Secret History of the War on Cancer*

Some of these dangerous molecules are obvious like smoking, while others may be new to you.

**Tobacco (smoked or chewed)**- Smoking or exposure to secondhand smoke can increase the risk of lung cancer, as well as many other types of cancer.

    **What to do**- Stop smoking, and avoid hanging out with others who smoke. Use the patch, hypnosis, and detox techniques as needed to stop smoking as soon as possible.

**Pesticides and herbicides**- These chemicals are often used in agriculture to kill insects and weeds, but they are also harmful to human health. Some pesticides and herbicides have been linked to cancer, and exposure to these chemicals should be minimized.

    **What to do**- Buy organic foods and produce when you can. If chemical sprays must be used, wear gloves, protective clothing, and a mask when spraying. Preferably, use natural, organic methods for insect control including: diatomaceous earth, boric acid, and essential oils.

**Asbestos**- This mineral was widely used in construction materials in the past, but it has been linked to lung cancer and mesothelioma. Asbestos is still present in many older buildings, so it's important to take precautions when renovating or demolishing these structures.

**What to do**- Generally, it is believed that as long as asbestos is left undisturbed in the insulation, then it will not get into the air and increase cancer risk. So if you have an old home with potential asbestos insulation around pipes etc, just don't disturb it, or get it professionally remediated if you can afford it.

**Benzene**- This chemical is used in the production of many products, including plastics, rubber, and detergents. It has been linked to leukemia and other types of cancer.

**What to do**- If you are an auto mechanic, professional painter, hobby painter, or regularly contact solvents, cleaners, gasoline, or paints, always wear plastic or rubber gloves to prevent benzene and other solvents from absorbing into the skin, and wear a carbon-filtered breathing mask if you're actively spraying or using concentrated chemicals with fumes.

**BPA & Phthalates**- are used in a variety of products, including toys, food packaging, personal care products (such as shampoo and lotion), thermal store receipts, and medical devices. They are known to be endocrine disruptors, which means they can interfere with the body's hormonal balance, which can contribute to cancer.

**What to do**- When you can, avoid drinking from plastic bottles, and never ever microwave food in or on plastic or styrofoam containers or food covered in plastic wrap. Wash your hands after handling store receipts.

**Parabens**- are a group of synthetic preservatives commonly used in cosmetics, personal care products, and food to prevent the growth of bacteria, mold, and yeast. There has been some concern that parabens may have estrogen-like effects on the body, which could potentially increase the risk of breast and other cancers.

**What to do-** Check ingredient labels and only purchase personal care products and cosmetics that are labeled paraben free. Personal care

products purchased from health food stores are generally safer, healthier, and more natural than those from standard grocery stores or malls.

**Synthetic flavors, colors & fragrances-** Artificial colors, flavors, and smells in foods, cosmetics, soaps, dryer sheets, and air fresheners, are generally not tested for safety alone or in combination with the 1000's of other chemicals in the environment. They have been linked to everything from cancer to asthma and ADHD.

**What to do-** If you want to minimize your exposure to synthetic fragrances, you can look for products that are labeled 'fragrance-free' or 'unscented.' Anything that says 'fragrance' or 'parfum' on the label is toxic. You can also choose products that use natural fragrances, such as essential oils or plant extracts, instead of synthetic fragrances. Choose only foods and cosmetics with natural colors and flavors. Avoid conventional perfumes and air fresheners, and use food-grade essential oils for fragrance on your body and in your home.

## Chapter 12 Action Steps

- If you live alone, have a friend come over and help you clean out your kitchen cupboards, closets, bathroom, and garage from all artificial or synthetic: cleaners, soaps, perfumes, cosmetics, sprays, air fresheners, solvents, pesticides, herbicides, etc.

- If you live in a family, have a family meeting and assign tasks to help overhaul your home and make it as free from synthetic chemicals as humanly possible.

- No one is perfect in this area, and we all probably have some synthetic products around. Do not let this exercise cause you more stress and frustration. Just put on some music and have fun purging and tossing out these artificial chemicals from your life, and then do

- the best you can to not bring them back into your home by using safer alternatives.
- Use organic and natural cosmetics, sunscreens, castile soap, and essential oils for cleaning. Hot water will clean most things. Essential oils of lemon or orange make great degreasers to break down stains, glues, and oil-based materials.

## Resources

### Books:

**Clean, Green, & Lean**   -Walter Crinnion

**The Secret History of the War on Cancer**   -Devra Davis

### Podcast:

**The Natural Cancer Support Channel- YouTube**

Podcast episodes with **Tee Forton Barnes** & **Amy Todisco**

# Chapter 13

## The Physical Pathway: Part 1 Exercise, Breathing & Fasting

"Exercise should be a part of the treatment plan for all cancer patients, no matter what stage or what diagnosis,"

-Dr Julie Gralow

Exercise and Fasting are the 2 most critical habits to use from the physical pathway. They can be miraculous when used alone, but when used in combination (not necessarily at the same time, but alternating) they can be an incredible anticancer force.

> **Exercise**- Trampoline, swimming, yoga, tai chi, qigong, and walking may be among the best exercises for cancer patients, but any and all movement is critical for cancer prevention and treatment. Many doctors have said something like: **"if I only had one therapy to use along with conventional cancer treatments, it would be exercise."**

If exercise were put into a bottle, and made available in pharmacies, it would become a trillion-dollar best-selling wonder drug. A study in 2017 stated,

**"We recently demonstrated that voluntary exercise leads to an influx of immune cells in tumors, and a more than 60% reduction in tumor incidence and growth across several mouse models."**

So we are learning that exercise is not just a nice thing to do to feel a little healthier when you have cancer, but it is actually a powerful cancer treatment itself.

**Here is a small sampling of quotations from medical research on cancer and exercise.**

"(yoga) has been shown to improve physical and mental health in people with different cancer types."

"(yoga) participants demonstrated significantly greater improvements in cancer related fatigue compared with participants in standard survivorship care at post-intervention."

"Walking is effective for cancer related fatigue during and after cancer therapy." (at least 6 weeks was more effective than fewer weeks of walking)

"Participating in more than 150 minutes per week of physical activity reduced lung cancer mortality."

"Cancer patients with moderate to severe cancer-related fatigue were significantly less in the Baduanjin (Qigong) group compared with the control group."

"Qigong therapy was found to have positive effects on the cancer-specific quality of life, fatigue, immune function, and cortisol levels of individuals with cancer."

**Exercise While On Oxygen Therapy (EWOT)-** is breathing oxygen through a special mask while on a treadmill or bike. Breathing O2 at a rate of 6 liters per minute, exercising for 30 minutes. Tumors are in a hypoxic (low oxygen) state and this makes them more aggressive and dangerous. So the theory is that oxygenating the entire body will help drive more oxygen into the cancer cells and reduce the aggressiveness of the tumor.

**Deep Breathing-** Deep breathing exercises can be helpful for supporting patients through conventional cancer treatments, as well as increasing life, health, and vitality in general. Deep breathing can help reduce stress and

anxiety, improve tissue oxygenation, support lymphatic function, enhance immune function, and improve mood.

**Fasting**- periodic fasting from all food for 1-4 days per month can help the digestive system rest and it supports healing in a number of ways. Fasting has been used for thousands of years in many spiritual and health practices throughout the world. Specifically for cancer, fasting has been studied to weaken cancer cells, strengthen normal cells, make cancer cells more susceptible to chemo and radiation, and dramatically reduce the side-effects from chemo and radiation. A research study stated that, "Fasting or fasting-mimicking diets (FMDs) lead to wide alterations in growth factors and in metabolite levels, generating environments that can reduce the capability of cancer cells to adapt and survive and thus improving the effects of cancer therapies."

Valter Longo PhD, Researcher at USC Norris Cancer Center, said, "Fasting makes it worse for cancer cells by generating an extreme environment with low glucose and growth factors and high ketone bodies, which weakens cancer cells. Each mutation in cancer cells makes them a little better at growing under standard conditions, but a little worse at surviving under extreme environments such as that caused by fasting".

**What to do**- It is best to be guided by a naturopathic doctor or clinical nutritionist who has experience with fasting and cancer, however if you cannot find one of these to work with, the basic principles for a 4-day fast before chemo or radiation are as follows:

1) For the 2 weeks before you are going to start a chemo or radiation treatment, increase vegetables, salads, and green smoothies for increased fiber and phytochemicals.

2) 3 days before the chemo or radiation treatment, ramp down calories by eating just 2 small lower-carb meals that day.

3) On the morning of 2 days before the cancer treatment, consume MCT Oil (liquid coconut oil) or supplemental ketones, then walk outside or on a treadmill for 3-4 hours while sipping water, vegetable broth (for minerals & electrolytes), and herbal teas. This

4) helps jump start your body into ketosis, or fat-burning mode. You can bring a companion to talk with, or listen to podcasts, or audiobooks during the long walk.

5) For the rest of the 4-day fast, consume purified water, herbal teas, and vegetable broth throughout the day. If you become too fatigued

or experience brain fog, consume more MCT oil or supplemental ketones as needed.

6) You will do this fast for 2 days before your treatment, and then the day of, and the day after the treatment.

7) On the 5th day, reintroduce foods slowly with easy to digest things like green smoothies, slow-cooked vegetables, and soups.

This is an ideal version of a fast. If it sounds too complicated, or if you are just not up for it. It can be simplified to just skipping solid food and drinking water, and broth, or green juice the day before you go in for the treatment, and the day of treatment.

Fasting can be life-changing in its ability to reduce side effects and weaken cancer cells to make conventional treatments more powerful.

# Chapter 13 Action Steps

1) Assess your exercise & activity levels. If you are very active and move a lot every day, congratulations! Move on to step number 2. If you know you need to increase your activity levels, brainstorm ways to increase your movement levels based on the following criteria:

- What physical activities or sports do you love to do?

- What kinds of play and movement did you enjoy as a child?

- What can you do in the season and climate you are in?

- What do you have the energy and time for?

- Do you have any pain, or other disability that requires modification of the amount and types of exercise you do?

- Take a timeout whenever you feel stressed, or before each meal, to do 10-20 deep belly breaths (outside in the fresh air for bonus points!)

2) If you are scheduled to have chemotherapy soon, plan out a fast on your calendar for a few days before each treatment starts.

3) If chemo is not currently recommended for you right now, plan out a 4-day fast on your calendar to weaken cancer cells, reboot your immune system, and adapt your body to burning fat (ketones) for fuel instead of glucose.

# Resources

## Books:

**Moving Through Cancer: An Exercise and Strength-Training Program for the Fight of Your Life**   -Dr. Kathryn Schmitz

**Tools of Titans**   -Tim Ferriss

## Exercise References:

Cramer H, Lauche R, Klose P, Lange S, Langhorst J, Dobos GJ. **Yoga for improving health-related quality of life, mental health and cancer-related symptoms in women diagnosed with breast cancer.** Cochrane Database Syst Rev. 2017 Jan 3;1(1):CD010802. doi: 10.1002/14651858.CD010802.pub2. PMID: 28045199; PMCID: PMC6465041.

Lin PJ, Kleckner IR, Loh KP, Inglis JE, Peppone LJ, Janelsins MC, Kamen CS, Heckler CE, Culakova E, Pigeon WR, Reddy PS, Messino MJ, Gaur R, Mustian KM. **Influence of Yoga on Cancer-Related Fatigue and on Mediational Relationships Between Changes in Sleep and Cancer-Related Fatigue: A Nationwide, Multicenter Randomized Controlled Trial of Yoga in Cancer Survivors.** Integr Cancer Ther. 2019 Jan-Dec;18:1534735419855134. doi: 10.1177/1534735419855134. PMID: 31165647; PMCID: PMC6552348.

Wang P, Wang D, Meng A, Zhi X, Zhu P, Lu L, Tang L, Pu Y, Li X. **Effects of Walking on Fatigue in Cancer Patients: A Systematic Review and Meta-analysis.** Cancer Nurs. 2022 Jan-Feb 01;45(1):E270-E278. doi: 10.1097/NCC.0000000000000914. PMID: 34870943.

Lee J. **Cardiorespiratory Fitness, Physical Activity, Walking Speed, Lack of Participation in Leisure Activities, and Lung Cancer Mortality: A Systematic Review and Meta-Analysis of Prospective Cohort Studies.** Cancer Nurs. 2021 Nov-Dec 01;44(6):453-464. doi: 10.1097/NCC.0000000000000847. PMID: 32590383.

Klein PJ, Schneider R, Rhoads CJ. **Qigong in cancer care: a systematic review and construct analysis of effective Qigong therapy.** Support Care Cancer. 2016 Jul;24(7):3209-22. doi: 10.1007/s00520-016-3201-7. Epub 2016 Apr 5. PMID: 27044279.

Kuo CC, Wang CC, Chang WL, Liao TC, Chen PE, Tung TH. **Clinical Effects of Baduanjin Qigong Exercise on Cancer Patients: A Systematic Review and Meta-Analysis on Randomized Controlled Trials.** Evid Based Complement Alternat Med. 2021 Apr 8;2021:6651238. doi: 10.1155/2021/6651238. PMID: 33880125; PMCID: PMC8049783.

# Fasting References:

Lettieri-Barbato D, Aquilano K. **Pushing the Limits of Cancer Therapy: The Nutrient Game.** Front Oncol. 2018 May 8;8:148. doi: 10.3389/fonc.2018.00148. PMID: 29868472; PMCID: PMC5951973.

Nencioni A, Caffa I, Cortellino S, Longo VD. **Fasting and cancer: molecular mechanisms and clinical application.** Nat Rev Cancer. 2018 Nov;18(11):707-719. doi: 10.1038/s41568-018-0061-0. PMID: 30327499; PMCID: PMC6938162.

Lee C, Raffaghello L, Brandhorst S, Safdie FM, Bianchi G, Martin-Montalvo A, Pistoia V, Wei M, Hwang S, Merlino A, Emionite L, de Cabo R, Longo VD. **Fasting cycles retard growth of tumors and sensitize a range of cancer cell types to chemotherapy.** Sci Transl Med. 2012 Mar 7;4(124):124ra27. doi: 10.1126/scitranslmed.3003293. Epub 2012 Feb 8. PMID: 22323820; PMCID: PMC3608686.

Saleh AD, Simone BA, Palazzo J, Savage JE, Sano Y, Dan T, Jin L, Champ CE, Zhao S, Lim M, Sotgia F, Camphausen K, Pestell RG, Mitchell JB, Lisanti MP, Simone NL. **Caloric restriction augments radiation efficacy in breast cancer.** Cell Cycle. 2013 Jun 15;12(12):1955-63. doi: 10.4161/cc.25016. Epub 2013 May 21. PMID: 23708519; PMCID: PMC3735710.

Simone BA, Palagani A, Strickland K, Ko K, Jin L, Lim MK, Dan TD, Sarich M, Monti DA, Cristofanilli M, Simone NL. **Caloric restriction counteracts chemotherapy-induced inflammation and increases response to therapy in a triple negative breast cancer model.** Cell Cycle. 2018;17(13):1536-1544. doi: 10.1080/15384101.2018.1471314. Epub 2018 Aug 6. PMID: 29912618; PMCID: PMC6133339.

# Chapter 14

## The Physical Pathway: Part 2 Other Physical Treatments

"Both earthing and grounding offer cancer patients a sense of empowerment and control over their health."

- Jodi Puhalla

**Castor Oil Packs**- Castor-oil packs are a staple of naturopathic medicine. Castor oil helps to detoxify the body, increase lymphatic circulation, decrease liver inflammation, and increase healthy colon function. For general health, the packs can be used over the liver (the right side of your lower rib cage) every night before bed. For faster healing from radiation therapy, you can use a castor oil pack over the treated area. Simply pour about 4 tablespoons of organic castor oil on a pad of cotton flannel and place it over the liver or irradiated area before bed. There are special reusable packs with ties that can be found on Amazon.com by searching "castor oil pack for liver". On following nights add 1-3 tablespoons of fresh oil to the pack each night so that it becomes more and more saturated as you go. You can take breaks from the castor oil packs 1 week out of every month, or 2 days out of every week if you would like.

**Clay Therapy**- Medicinal clay has the power to support the healing of tissues from radiation burns and can be an integral part of healing after radiation therapy. Clay can also be used internally and externally for detoxification of heavy metals, pesticides, environmental pollution, etc. There are many different types of clay such as French Green Clay, Bentonite Clay, and Aztec Clay. You can purchase powdered medicinal clay from most health food stores or online. The powdered clay is then gradually mixed with water until it has a paste-like consistency. The clay can then be applied to any area of the body, just avoid the eyes and other sensitive areas as the clay can be a bit abrasive when washing it off. Spread the clay over the desired area and then let it dry and leave on for 20-60 minutes. Then wash it off in the sink or shower. You can also take clay baths sprinkling 1 cup of powdered clay into your bath and stirring until dissolved. Shower off the clay residue after the bath.

**Earthing / Grounding-** Earthing is the simple act of touching the earth with your bare feet and hands. There are similarities between the earth's magnetic and electric fields and the fields of your brain and heart. By physically connecting to the earth, you electrically ground your body so that surplus electrons flow into the earth. Or, if you are deficient in electrons, the earth can supply you with the electrical balance that you need. This is free and easy to do, just take off your shoes and walk and play in the lawn or a park more often.

**Massage therapy-** Just like exercise, massage therapy provides mechanical stress to the tissues and this increases circulation, oxygenation, and pain relief to the area. Lymphatic massage is a specialty that some massage therapists offer, and is the most specific for cancer recovery. Massage is also a great way to apply healing massage oils and essential oils described in the molecular pathway directly to the body. Dr Christopher, a prominent American herbalist from the 1950's-1980's taught a special 3 oil massage as part of his "incurables" program. "For the first two days, massage the patient with castor oil, using a clockwise circular motion from the top of the head to the bottom of the feet, always working towards the heart. The next two days use olive oil, and the last two days of the week massage with wheat germ oil." These simple, nourishing treatments can have powerful additive effects when combined with a total healing program.

**Reflexology-** is an easy at-home treatment that consists of pressing on certain points on the body that can stimulate the nerves connected to certain organs to create greater health and balance throughout the body. There are specific reflexology charts for the hands, feet, and body. You can find charts in books or through an online image search. This is free, easy, and has no side-effects, so I recommend giving it a try for pain, nausea, or other symptoms you may be experiencing.

**Acupressure**- Is very similar to reflexology, but it applies pressure to the traditional Chinese acupuncture points found all over the body. This is more involved and advanced than reflexology because it employs over 360 specific body points, so seeing a professional acupressure practitioner may be an easier option.

**Joint Manipulation**- Alignment and posture of the spine and other joints can relieve pain, stress, and pressure on the various nerves that provide healing signals to and from the brain and spinal cord. Chiropractors, Osteopaths, and Naturopathic Doctors all have training in these special joint manipulations.

**Hydrotherapy**- Is the use of temperature and water to affect changes in circulation and other bodily functions. Some of the most effective treatments include:

- **Contrast Showers**- One of the most simple and powerful hydrotherapy remedies is the hot and cold contrast shower. This treatment is great for morning fatigue, aches and pains, or simply lifting your mood. As most people in our society already take showers everyday, this habit takes no extra time or money out of your life.

  In the shower, simply turn the water to as hot as you can stand without causing pain or burning for about 1 minute, then turn the temperature to cool or cold for about 30 seconds, then turn back to hot for 1 minute, then back to cool for 30 seconds, and do anywhere from 3 to 6 alternations of hot and cold. This may be challenging at first, but try to take some deep breaths while you turn it to cold, and allow your body to surrender to the sensations!

  The powerful contrast brings blood flow to the surface of your skin when sprayed with hot water, and blood flow is driven to the core of the body when sprayed with cold water. So in 6 minutes or less you can have the equivalent of a full-body workout of blood circulation. It's not the extreme temperatures that matter as much as the contrast, so if you are feeling weak, or it's the middle of winter, a warm and cool contrast can be an effective substitute for the more extreme hot and cold contrast shower. Studies show that contrast showers can improve muscle soreness and reduce pain. I promise that if you make this simple remedy a habit, it will change your life for the better!

- **Epsom Salt Baths**- Epsom salt is the common name for magnesium sulfate crystals. This means that it is made of magnesium, sulfur, and oxygen atoms. Magnesium is one of the main "relaxation" minerals and one of the most important and often deficient minerals in the human body; sulfur strengthens connective tissue, and aids in liver detoxification. When Epsom salt is dissolved in a hot bath, it can promote muscle relaxation, cellular detoxification, and pain relief.

- **Foot Baths**- Using a hot foot bath can draw more blood flow out of the head when you have a pounding headache. Medicated foot baths are essentially soaking your feet in herbal tea. This is especially useful for nausea when undergoing chemo or radiation. If you can't keep anything down, you can soak your feet in herbal tea to calm the nerves and reduce nausea. Herbs like ginger, cinnamon, and peppermint are good choices.

- **Constitutional Hydrotherapy**- Is a very powerful treatment using alternating hot and cold towels on your back and chest combined with electrical stimulation to specific nerve areas on the abdomen and back. This is available at the teaching clinics of Naturopathic medical schools and at many private Naturopathic practices throughout the US and Canada.

- **Colon Cleansing**- The colon is the number one pathway the body uses to eliminate toxic substances from our internal and external environments. When going through a detoxification program, extra toxins are flowing into the colon. If you have any level of constipation or sluggish bowel movements, the toxins can then be
- reabsorbed into the bloodstream making you feel even more sick. Through the use of enemas or colon hydrotherapy, you can eliminate these toxic molecules before they can cause any more harm.

**Forest Bathing-** Forest bathing, also known as Shinrin-yoku, is a practice that originated in Japan in the 1980s and involves spending time in nature, particularly in forests, to improve one's overall well-being. The practice has gained popularity worldwide and has been the subject of several scientific studies.

The science of forest bathing involves the study of the physiological and psychological effects of spending time in nature, particularly in forests. Research has shown that spending time in nature can have a positive impact on stress reduction, immune system function, blood pressure, mood, and overall sense of well-being.

One of the many key medicinal components of forest bathing is the exposure to terpenes, which are the volatile organic compounds emitted into the air by trees and plants. These compounds have been shown to have anti-inflammatory, anti-tumor, and antimicrobial effects, which may contribute to the health benefits of spending time in forests.

## Chapter 14 Action Steps

1) Take note of which 1 or 2 therapies appealed to you the most. If you have radiation burns, use castor oil packs and clay packs alternating every other day. As often as you can, get out into the forest and breathe deeply. Walk barefoot in the grass whenever you have the chance. Mark your calendar for your next massage or acupressure session. Select the actions that bring you joy, and help you feel the most nurtured, and most connected to the earth and others.

## Resources

### Books:

**The Oil That Heals** -William A. & M.D. McGarey

**Healing with Clay** -Ran Knishinsky

**Earthing: The Most Important Health Discovery Ever**

– Clinton Ober Dr Stephen Sinatra, & Martin Zucker

**Body Reflexology: Healing at Your Fingertips**
–Mildred Carter & Tammy Weber

**Forest Bathing: How Trees Can Help You Find Health and Happiness**
–Dr. Qing Li

## Websites:

https://www.herballegacy.com/Three_Oil_Massage.html

# Chapter 15

## The Genetic Pathway

"Epigenetics doesn't change the genetic code, it changes how it's read."

-Bruce Lipton author of, *The Biology of Belief*

This chapter offers optional information that may be helpful in customizing treatments.

Warning: if you are not a science geek, this pathway may be too overwhelming, and become too much of a complex rabbit hole to explore. If you would rather just focus on living your life and getting better, then feel free to skip this pathway.

However, if you love science and health, and are excited to learn more about ways to customize your lifestyle to match your unique genetic makeup, then the rabbit hole awaits...

**Genetics vs. Epigenetics-** An important point to understand is the difference between genetics and epigenetics. Genetics refers to your actual DNA code, and epigenetics refers to how that DNA code is read and expressed. This is what people mean when they refer to genes being turned on or turned off. In reality, genes don't turn off or on, it is more like they are covered or uncovered. When a gene is not being expressed it is coiled around a protein called a histone (Think of DNA as the string and a histone as the yo-yo). When the DNA string is unwrapped from around the yo-yo it can be read and copied, and when the string is wrapped tightly around the histone/yo-yo it cannot be read or expressed. Methylation, or adding a methyl group to the DNA or the histone, is one of the main regulators of gene expression. The bottom line of what epigenetics means to us as individuals, is that your genes are not your destiny. If you have "bad" genes combined with a healthy lifestyle then you will still be able to express your genes in a healthy way, and if you have good genes and a

terrible lifestyle, you can still shorten your life. It is important to remember that almost all of the pathways that we have discussed so far can influence the epigenetic expression of your genes. So if you do DNA testing, and it tells you that you have higher risks of certain conditions, just know that the more healthy changes you make, the lower your will risks become.

**DNA testing and interpretation**- 23andMe has the most affordable genetic testing I know about. You can run the results through different websites to learn more about your genetic strengths and weaknesses, and how to customize your supplements, medications, and lifestyle.

Some of the major genes that create enzymes that are involved in the cancer process include:

**Methylenetetrahydrofolate reductase (MTHFR)**- is an enzyme that plays a crucial role in the metabolism of folate (Vitamin B-9) and the regulation of DNA methylation. Genetic mutations in the MTHFR gene can affect the activity of the enzyme, leading to changes in folate metabolism and DNA methylation patterns. Research suggests that MTHFR mutations may be associated with an increased risk of certain types of cancer, including colorectal cancer, breast cancer, and leukemia.

**Glutathione S-transferase (GST)**- This family of genes encodes a group of enzymes that play a critical role in the detoxification of dangerous environmental chemicals, including carcinogens. Certain genetic variations in the GST genes can result in reduced or altered enzyme activity, which may affect an individual's ability to remove harmful substances from the body.

Studies have suggested that these genetic variations in the GST genes may be associated with an increased risk of cancer, particularly in individuals

who are exposed to environmental toxins or who have a family history of cancer. Additionally, some cancer treatments, such as chemotherapy and radiation can increase the production of reactive oxygen species, which may be detoxified by GST enzymes. Thus, genetic variations in the GST genes may also impact the effectiveness and toxicity of cancer treatments.

Learning about mutations that you have in this set of genes may help you and your oncologist make decisions about the dosing and frequency of chemotherapy. If you are a fast metabolizer of the particular drug, then you may need a higher dose in your system for it to be effective because your body clears it out so fast. And, if you are a slow metabolizer, the toxic drug will stay in your system longer, so you can have a good therapeutic effect with a lower dose and potentially have fewer side effects.

**Catechol-o-methyl-transferase (COMT)-** is an enzyme that adds a methyl group (one carbon atom attached to 3 hydrogen atoms) to a molecule to activate or transform it. This relates to cancer in a few ways. Estrogens are metabolized into various downstream versions that can have either procarcinogenic potential or anticarcinogenic potential. 2 Methoxy estradiol is a very cancer protective version of estrogen, and as the name implies it has a methyl group attached to it by the COMT enzyme. The issue is that COMT also adds a methyl group to create adrenaline molecules from noradrenaline, So if we are under chronic stress and are needing to synthesize extra adrenaline the COMT enzyme will be busy activating adrenaline, and will be too occupied to transform the more cancer promoting estradiol into the healthy cancer protective 2 methoxy estradiol. This is one of the biochemical reasons that stress is more cancer-promoting. Through genetic testing, you can find out if you have an efficient or a sluggish COMT enzyme. Then, with the help of your doctor, you can make needed adjustments to optimize your methylation levels.

**Phosphatidylethanolamine N-methyltransferase (PEMT)-** gene encodes an enzyme that plays a crucial role in the production of phosphatidylcholine, a major component of cell membranes. Research has suggested that alterations in PEMT gene expression may be associated with cancer development and progression.

Studies have shown that high levels of PEMT expression are correlated with poor outcomes in certain types of cancer, such as breast, ovarian, and pancreatic cancer. Conversely, low levels of PEMT expression have been associated with better outcomes in some types of cancer, including hepatocellular carcinoma. It is thought that alterations in PEMT expression may impact cell proliferation, apoptosis, and other cellular processes that are important for cancer development and progression.

### Now Let's Take a Look at a Few of the Major Oncogenes (Cancer Genes) and Cell Signaling Molecules

**Oncogenes-** are genes that have the potential to cause cancer when they are mutated or overexpressed. Normally, oncogenes are involved in regulating cell growth and division, but when they are mutated, they can promote uncontrolled cell growth and division, leading to the development and progression of cancer.

Targeting oncogenes is a promising area of cancer therapy, and several drugs have been developed that specifically target the products of oncogenes or the pathways that they regulate. An example of this is the drug Herceptin, which helps block the effects of the Her2/neu gene. By targeting oncogenes, it may be possible to slow or stop the growth of cancer cells while minimizing the side effects of treatment.

**P53-** This is a tumor suppressor gene that plays a critical role in preventing the development and progression of cancer. It is often called the "guardian of the genome" because of its ability to monitor and repair DNA damage, and to induce apoptosis (programmed cell death) in cells that have sustained irreparable damage. Mutations in the p53 gene are among the most common genetic alterations found in cancer. When the p53 gene is mutated or absent, cells may be unable to repair DNA damage properly, leading to the accumulation of mutations and the development of cancer.

So increased P53 activity is a good thing, and we want to increase P53 in our cells. By following a balanced program based on the 7 Pathways, you can increase your P53 naturally.

**RAS-** This family of 36 known genes is important for cell signaling pathways that regulate cell growth, differentiation, and survival. Mutations in RAS genes are among the most common genetic alterations found in cancer, and they can lead to the development and progression of several types of cancer, including lung, colon, and pancreatic cancer. Mutated RAS genes can promote uncontrolled cell growth and division, inhibit apoptosis, and promote tumor angiogenesis, which allows tumors to obtain nutrients and oxygen from surrounding tissues. Although RAS mutations are extremely common in cancer, they have been challenging to target with cancer therapies due to their complex signaling pathways. However, researchers continue to study RAS biology and search for new approaches to target RAS-driven cancers.

**BCL-** These proteins play an important role in regulating apoptosis and their dysregulation is implicated in the development and progression of cancer. Some members of the BCL family, such as BCL-2, promote cancer cell survival by inhibiting apoptosis, while other members, such as BAX and BAK, promote apoptosis by disrupting the integrity of mitochondrial membranes. So it is the balance between pro-apoptotic (good guy) and anti-apoptotic (bad guy) BCL proteins that is important.. The overexpression of anti-apoptotic BCL proteins, such as BCL-2, is commonly observed in cancer and can contribute to treatment resistance. So we want lower BCL-2 and higher BAX & BAK, and ways to do this are constantly being studied.

**VEGF-** Vascular Endothelial Growth Factor is a signaling protein that plays a key role in the growth of new blood vessels, or angiogenesis. In cancer, VEGF can be overexpressed, promoting the growth of new blood vessels to supply the tumor with nutrients and oxygen. Blocking VEGF signaling has become an important target for cancer therapy, and several drugs have been developed that target VEGF or its receptor to inhibit angiogenesis and starve tumors of their blood supply. Many of the foods and herbs covered in the molecular pathway help inhibit angiogenesis by blocking or lowering VEGF.

**BRCA-** These are the infamous genes that have caused women to have prophylactic double mastectomies when mutations in these genes are found. BRCA1 and BRCA2 are tumor suppressor genes that play a critical role in DNA repair. Inherited mutations in these genes cause them to work more slowly, and are associated with an increased risk of developing breast, ovarian, and other types of cancer. Mutations in BRCA genes can result in an accumulation of genetic damage and increase the risk of cells becoming cancerous. Genetic testing can identify BRCA mutations, and individuals with a family history of cancer may be advised to undergo testing to assess their risk. A challenging difference between The philosophies of conventional medicine versus naturopathic medicine is that with a BRCA mutation a woman is more susceptible to the genetic damage to DNA from things such as x-rays. So as a naturopathic physician, I would recommend a patient with this mutation to not have routine mammograms, and only use a combination of physical breast exams, ultrasound, MRI, and thermography for safer breast cancer screenings. Conventional medicine however, often recommends more frequent mammograms for women with a family history of breast cancer or a known BRCA mutation. I believe this is dangerous and the combination of smashing pressure and x-rays can increase the risk of developing breast cancer in women with these BRCA differences.

**MTOR-** is an enzyme that plays a crucial role in regulating cell growth, metabolism, and survival. It has been found that MTOR is frequently deregulated in cancer cells, leading to uncontrolled cell proliferation and survival. MTOR activation promotes tumor growth and progression by increasing protein synthesis, cell cycle progression, and angiogenesis. Therefore, MTOR inhibitors have been developed as a promising therapeutic strategy for cancer treatment, particularly for those with MTOR pathway dysregulation.

## Chapter 15 Action Steps

1) If you are interested in learning more about your genetics, order a Health + Ancestry test kit from www.23andme.com for about $200.

2) When you have sent in your sample and have your results back, you select "browse raw data" under your account profile tab, then click "download" at the top, center, 2nd menu down.

3) This allows you to upload your raw DNA file to other websites such as: Nebula Genomics, Genetic Genie, or Genome Link.

4) It is definitely recommended that you work with a Naturopathic or Functional Medicine Doctor who has some training in genomics to understand your individual results and how to apply them to your life.

# Resources

**Books:**

**Dirty Genes** -Dr. Ben Lynch

**The Biology of Belief** -Dr. Bruce Lipton

**Websites:**

https://www.23andme.com

https://nebula.org

https://geneticgenie.org

https://genomelink.io

# Chapter 16

## The Social Pathway

"What matters in the circle of the Cancer Help Program is that we share a wound, and that we are brothers and sisters; we are beloved of each other in that circle."

–Michael Lerner

As humans we are social beings, the better our social connections to family and friends, the more happy and healthy we will generally be. Studies have shown that people with the lowest levels of social support had immune systems that did not function as well. A number of studies have also correlated loneliness with unusually high incidences of cancer. Consider these Social Pathway options.

**Choosing a Cancer Advocate**- It is recommended that you choose a family member or friend to be an advocate for you. This will be someone who can attend doctor visits with you, hold your hand, offer hugs, help with research, and make sure your questions at appointments get asked and answered, and notes are taken.

**Family gatherings**- Family gatherings can be a powerful and beautiful source of healing and joy, but the flip side is that you can also trigger old memories and stresses. Only you know if family gatherings will be a part of your healing journey or not. But if not, this is a sign that greater social and emotional healing needs to take place through conversations, forgiveness, family therapy, or other tools. Schedule more time to be with your family members that are uplifting, fun, and joyful, and spend less time with family members who cause extra stress and drama in your life.

**Fun and Laughter with Friends**- Sharing a meal, playing games, lively group conversation, these can be some of the most beautiful moments of life where all of our depressions, anxieties, and pains melt away. It is almost always better to laugh with family or friends than all by yourself. Planning for these moments, either long distance through video chat, or

in-person gatherings can be an important part of using the social pathway for healing.

**Group Therapy-** Dr David Spiegel unexpectedly found that women who participated in a support group lived almost twice as long as those that did not. Many other studies have confirmed this finding. Group therapy can be life changing for cancer patients, or if a family or work dynamic is causing chronic pain and stress. There are two types of group therapy; one is a support group format with a trained counselor moderator leading a group of individuals who don't know each other, but face a similar challenge such as cancer, anxiety, or chronic pain. The other is with a group that you know such as friends, family, or business associates. The counselor helps make sure that everyone is heard, works on the group dynamic, and helps balance the individual and group goals.

**Family Therapy-** If your family is not in harmony with your medical choices for cancer treatment, or your family pattern of stress, pain, and trauma is adding a burden to your life, then family therapy can help sort out the patterns of pain and stress, and lead to eventual healing.

**Couples Therapy-** A spouse or life partner has the most profound influence on our physical and emotional health of any other person besides ourselves. If you are experiencing cancer combined with marital difficulties, your healing will generally be much more difficult. If your marriage relationship is a source of constant stress and emotional wounding, then professional support with a trained Marriage and Family Therapist (MFT) is the best idea. Couples counseling is sometimes covered by insurance plans, and if affordability is an issue, then therapy interns who charge a small cash fee while they are completing their training can be a good option.

**Social Meetups and Clubs-** Clubs, societies, and meetups can be a great place to meet new people, share information with other passionate like-minded people, and get out and explore the joy of learning and having

new experiences. Meetup.com, Craigslist.org, Facebook groups, and other similar sites are great ways of connecting with like-minded people who have an interest in similar topics or activities.

**Church Groups-** Church groups have the combined benefit of powerful spiritual connection and healing, as well as social network building and community. If you have a former faith you have drifted from, or have never quite found the best match for you, I would encourage you to return, or to search for a faith-based community that resonates with you. Church groups can provide a quality of love, empathy, support, faith, and prayer that regular clubs or support groups will never be able to match.

## Chapter 16 Action Steps

1) Choose someone who is willing to be your cancer advocate.

2) Spend as much quality time with family and friends as possible.

3) Research cancer support groups in your area and attend one. If you enjoy it, continue to go on a regular basis

4) If you desire more social connection, seek out clubs, meetups, or church groups that resonate with you.

5) If you have any unresolved conflicts in your marriage or family, seek couples or family counseling.

# Chapter 17

## The Spiritual Pathway

"Faith is the bird that sings when the dawn is still dark."

– Rabindranath Tagore

The goal of cancer treatment is not to prevent death because we will all die someday. The goal is to live better and live longer. These spiritual pathway goals help us to live in a way that results in happiness and peace of mind for us and those around us. Some have been studied scientifically and some have been simply accepted as healthy and powerful through thousands of years of traditional use.

**Purpose**- Critical questions to ponder are, "What is my life's purpose? Why am I here? What was I born to do?" By reflecting on these questions, you can craft and write a personal mission or vision statement. There are countless ways that connecting to your reason for living provides a powerful anchor and motivation to do all of the work required to travel down the seven pathways of healing. Life is hard; there are always challenges and setbacks along the way. By connecting with, and focusing energy on, your central life purposes, you can have the strength to get back up every time you fall. You will develop the long-term vision needed to try again every time you fail, and the courage to put one foot in front of the other, and take one more breath even when times are hardest.

**Values**- By going through a values clarification process, you can gain critical insights into what is in balance and out of balance with your own life values. If you have deeply-held values that you are not truly investing in with your time and energy, then your subconscious mind may give your body symptoms such as depression, anxiety, upset stomach, chronic pain, or other physical ailments. The more we can live in alignment with our own chosen set of values the more whole and healed our life will be.

Values are usually single words or short phrases such as family, learning, financial success, contribution, adventure, creativity, etc. These are aspects of life that you value; that are most valuable to your life and happiness. A values clarification exercise simply consists of brainstorming 6-12 of these values that come to mind, then coming up with a sentence, or short paragraph, that defines what that word means to you. Then sequencing these values in order of highest priority at the top of the list to lowest priority at the bottom. Then you have a sequenced list of values that are all important to you, but in order of priority with the highest priority at the top. Type out this list, print out several copies to put in various places like your bathroom mirror, as a bookmark in a book you're reading, or any other important place where you'll see it and read it often. Then consider your time and energy and how much of each you are devoting to each value.

You should generally be devoting the most concentrated effort toward your number-one value. Values are dynamic, and every day is different, so nothing is clean, orderly, or perfect in life. So give yourself lots of grace and forgiveness with this process, but by pursuing a path that continually strives to put more and more time and energy into the values that are most important to you, and less energy and time into the values that are least important, or that are not even values at all, I believe physical symptoms can heal much more quickly, and emotional symptoms can be transformed as well. A great book that provides a variation on this values clarification exercise is called *The Passion Test*, by Chris and Janet Attwood.

**Goals**- Goals are a fantastic tool to take the invisible world and make it visible. By setting goals that are in alignment with your purpose and your values, you can create a written list that you are pursuing, that can bring excitement, motivation, and joy to each and every day. The differences between purpose, values, and goals, are that your purpose and values are generally permanent, or at least change very slowly. They are never completed. They are like your compass; true north is always north. Once you decide and understand your purpose, it's a single statement to drive and motivate your entire life, but a goal, by definition, is a dream with a deadline, or a specific outcome that you intend to reach by a certain date.

In considering goals, there should be a balance between short-term, mid-range, and long-term goals, as well as a balance between physical, mental, spiritual, financial, relationship, and adventure goals etc. Nearly all experts on goals agree that it is best to start with a pure brainstorming session where you don't edit any ideas. Just write down as many ideas as you possibly can, at least 100 life goals is a good place to start. At this first stage, it is not edited for quality, and also some of these can be rather outlandish, or silly, or impractical, but this first step is more of an exercise in raw creativity and writing speed. In the context of healing from cancer, it is important to set physical goals that will be exciting and motivating for you to achieve in the future. Next, beside each goal write a preliminary date by which you plan to accomplish it. Then you can begin to sort and categorize this major list of goals into physical, mental, spiritual, financial categories, and sequence them in chronological order of accomplishment. You can start to shape this list into two separate lists; one for goals that you will be currently taking action on, and another list for "someday goals" that would be fun to accomplish in the far future, or that are impractical right now, but you would still like to hold on to them in a list for the future. The next part is up to you; you can create a horizontal timeline of the chronological order of all your future goal accomplishments, or write out all your accomplishment dates on a traditional paper calendar, or on your digital calendaring system. Any goal with complexity can be broken down into smaller monthly, weekly, and daily steps to provide for greater simplicity and clarity. Then, in the beginning of your monthly and weekly planning and calendaring, you can review the steps and goals you plan to accomplish that week, and review your list of values to make sure that your plans and goals are in alignment with your purpose and values. By connecting your daily and weekly actions to your values and purpose, you will ensure that you are investing your time in the things that matter most to you. By daily working to achieve goals that you have personally set in all areas of your life, you can gradually increase motivation, health, wellness, and joy in every category of your life.

**Legacy**- Legacy is thinking about the difference that you want to make in the world, and what you want to be remembered for after you're gone. This can start with the famous "tombstone" or "eulogy" exercise where you think about and attend your own funeral before you die in your

imagination. What would you want written on your tombstone? What would you want to have said about you at your funeral? What do you want to be remembered for? What have you accomplished? What relationships were most important to you? What charities did you start or contribute to? What causes did you champion? By pondering and journaling on the answers to these questions, it can inspire new thoughts and ideas to add to your goals list, and give you the long-term perspective that you need to live most effectively in "the now".

**Love**- Love, charity, goodwill, compassion, kindness, these are values that have been taught and embraced by all great spiritual traditions of the world. They are also the most universal positive emotions that we can experience. By contemplating the various aspects of love, how you can be more in alignment with universal love, and how you can take daily actions that are motivated by love, you can transform your life from the inside out. Just like turning on a flashlight in a dark room, love can instantly negate pain, fear, bitterness, frustration, apathy, and hate. If you let love be the theme and the driving force behind all of your goals, values, and purpose, then healing can be accelerated in every area of your life.

**Service**- Service is the magical elixir that allows us to transcend our own pain by focusing on helping, lifting, and relieving the pain of others. There are so many causes, so many nonprofits, and so many websites that list available opportunities for service, that the options are nearly endless. There are service opportunities for every level of skill, talent, age, or physical ability. It could be helping a neighbor rake leaves, reading to the blind, volunteering at a homeless shelter, or sewing blankets for refugees, the specific activity doesn't matter as much as your desire to give, and that it is a cause that resonates with your heart. We all know the story of *A Christmas Carol* with the dynamic character of Ebenezer Scrooge. There is the first part of his life spent in selfish misery, but in the final scenes he is transformed by service, contribution, and thinking of others instead of himself. He was able to let go of a lifetime of pain and misery, and

experience the joy of selflessness for the rest of his days. If regular service to others is not already a part of your life, I invite you to explore some of the many opportunities and causes to which you can contribute to make the world a better place.

**Gratitude**- "Thank you" is one of the great magical words we try to teach our toddlers in their first years of life. Gratitude and thanksgiving have such power to focus our love and emotions on the present moment, on what is good, on what is beautiful, and on what is working in our lives. As addressed in the emotional pathway section, science has proven that thoughts and emotions create new chemistry in our brains and bodies.

By focusing on gratitude in meditation, prayer, journaling, writing thank you letters, or in just saying thank you, you shift attention away from what is wrong, and toward what is right, and what you desire. This creates a positive upward spiral of better thoughts, emotions, and biochemistry. There is a saying that says, "pain is necessary, but suffering is optional". Gratitude is a force that can decrease suffering and increase joy when you make it a daily part of your life.

**Forgiveness**- Forgiveness is a double-sided coin; there are many things that we need to forgive that others have done to us, and there are many things that we need to ask others forgiveness for. There is a common saying that "holding a grudge is like drinking poison and expecting the other person to get sick." Holding back forgiveness from old hurts and deep wounds only makes those wounds go deeper and last longer. A great exercise is to pick up your journal, a loose sheet of paper, or your laptop, and brainstorm a list of those people from childhood onward who may have hurt, offended, or wounded you. After you are done making this list, go through each person one by one, close your eyes, imagine their face, and say something like: "I forgive you. It's okay now, I no longer hold any ill-will toward you. I may not agree with what you did, but I want to extend grace and forgiveness toward you to make the world a better place." Obviously, you can make up your own words and ideas customized to your situation.

Put a star by any of these individual's names that you feel you need to talk to over the phone, or in person, to extend forgiveness. For the next list, you write down the names of anyone that you believe you have, or may have, hurt, wounded, or offended. If it is someone that you no longer have contact with, or is no longer alive, simply think of their face and say to yourself, "I'm sorry, please forgive me." Again, put a star next to those for whom you know it is best to have an in-person conversation with to ask for forgiveness.

So often, it is those closest to us that are the easiest to hurt. Our parents, siblings, spouses, children, other family, and close friends are often the most in need of offering and asking for forgiveness. By focusing on both sides of the coin of asking for forgiveness, and offering forgiveness to others, you will begin to embody the concept behind the old song, "Let There Be Peace On Earth, and Let It Begin With Me."

**Faith**- Faith is one of the greatest powers in the universe. The power of faith, belief, or expectation is what drives us to wake up in the morning, to turn on the ignition in our car, to set goals, to plant seeds, to visit a doctor's office, to have children, or to take any other action. Faith is the power to use imagination to bring things out of the unseen world and into the seen world. Use the power of faith to believe in your physical healing, use your imagination to create a perfect blueprint of every organ and body part, whole, healed, and healthy. See its ideal, optimal, functioning state, with every organ system playing its part in the grand symphony that is your body and mind.

By increasing the power of your faith, you automatically decrease doubt, fear, and anxiety. Faith is the force that creates the future that you will step into tomorrow. By using intention to focus that faith to see the things that you truly desire, you will be creating a domino effect of greater tomorrows every day that you live.

Generally, I recommend only working with doctors and other practitioners who use therapies that you believe in and trust will work for you. Your belief gives power to whatever treatment you choose to undergo.

I have researched, but have still not been able to determine whether the following story is true, or if it is just urban legend, but I believe the principles behind it are absolutely true.

**Story**- "Many doctors know the story of "Mr. Wright," who was found to have cancer and in 1957 was given only days to live. Hospitalized in Long Beach, CA, with tumors the size of oranges, he heard that scientists had discovered a serum, called Krebiozen, that appeared to be effective against cancer. He begged to receive it.

His physician, Dr. Philip West, finally agreed and gave Mr. Wright an injection on a Friday afternoon. The following Monday, the astonished doctor found his patient out of his "death bed," joking with the nurses. The tumors, the doctor wrote later, "had melted like snowballs on a hot stove."

Two months later, Mr. Wright read medical reports that the serum was a quack remedy. He suffered an immediate relapse. "Don't believe what you read in the papers," the doctor told Mr. Wright. Then he injected him with what he said was "a new super-refined double strength" version of the drug. Actually, it was water, but again, the tumor masses melted.

Mr. Wright was "the picture of health" for another two months -- until he read a definitive report stating that Krebiozen was worthless. He died two days later."

This story illustrates the stunning power of our positive beliefs (placebo effect), and negative beliefs (nocebo effect) over life and death. Use your intention to focus your faith on your desired outcome. Your expectation contributes to your destiny; so expect the best, and then align your actions with that expectation.

**Intuition**- Learning to listen to your "inner knowing" or "the still small voice" when it comes to making choices is one of the most valuable skills anyone can learn. If you feel that a certain cancer therapy is right or wrong for you, then trust those feelings. Your inner compass has much more wisdom than many of us realize.

**Prayer**- Prayer is the act of focusing thought, gratitude, and intention toward the Creator. For billions of people around the world, prayer is a daily practice that increases purpose, meaning, and joy in their lives. Prayer is able to organize nearly all of the elements of the spiritual pathway together into one cohesive practice. We can pray to understand our purpose and values, and the best goals for us at the time, and then pray to live our purpose, values, and achieve those goals on a daily basis. We can pray for opportunities to increase love and service, and offer prayers of pure gratitude. By exercising faith in the things that we pray for, we add the power of visualization and mental effort to the process.

Dr. Larry Dossey and many others have researched the power of prayer scientifically. In double-blind studies, where those who were praying did not know exactly who they were praying for, and patients in hospitals who were prayed for did not know whether they were being prayed for or not, results have shown a healing power of prayer far beyond random chance. First, pray in gratitude for all that is going right in your life, and in your health, then ask for and see the ideal blueprint of your health and ask for the healing that you desire for yourself and others. Prayer can be a profound practice that will connect you to The Divine, to your highest self, and to the rest of your human family.

**Other Spiritual Healing**- There are countless spiritual and religious rituals that can assist in healing including: the laying on of hands, singing, shamanic journeys, the chanting and drumming of African or Native American healing traditions, and more. Just about every traditional culture has ancient wisdom for healing that can be studied and utilized as part of a healing path. As long as you develop a holistic treatment plan that includes all six or seven pathways of healing, and use common sense in avoiding things that could be hazardous to your health, these practices can magnify your faith and activate the innate healing response in your body which is the most powerful and desirable form of healing that you can experience. For too long, science has tried to downplay the placebo effect as something annoying to rule out of their research, or to downplay as non-scientific. However, the truth is that the placebo effect is the truest form of medicinethat exists. It is the unseen force within your body connecting with the unseen forces of the universe to provide pure healing.

It has been proven that the placebo effect actually causes healing molecules to be produced and circulated by the body. Endorphins are powerful morphine-like chemicals that the body creates in response to the power of belief to relieve pain. The opiate-blocking drug Narcan can actually be used to block this placebo pain-relieving effect. This proves that the placebo effect is not just wishful thinking, or mind over matter, but it is truly mind creating matter that can be blocked or measured in objective ways. The placebo effect is so important for your healing, that I believe it's essential that you choose treatments in each of these pathways that you believe in. Find the techniques that you have hope, faith, and trust in. Then find the healthcare professionals that you like and trust, that have good reviews, and good reputations. In my personal and professional experience, the seven pathways have the potential to absolutely transform your life and health for the better.

## Moving Along the 7 Pathways

While I tried to be as comprehensive as possible in listing the ideas and techniques available in each pathway, due to the time and space constraints of this book, I'm quite certain that there are hundreds of amazing ancient and cutting-edge therapies that I have missed covering here. As with so many things in life, the choice is yours. A book is only as effective as you make it.

Much motivation, faith, dedication, and persistence is required to achieve what others may perceive as a healing miracle. As you move forward along the pathways, you will learn that miracles can also be outcomes that you earn through taking action, creating healing habits, and thinking and working with a holistic framework to utilize the physical, molecular, emotional, spiritual, genetic, energetic, and social pathways of healing. With conventional medicine, the more doctors you see and the more medications you take, usually the more sick you will become because of the overlapping side effects of each medication. If you are taking more than one or two medications, this is probably too many and you should

work with your primary care doctor or other licensed medical professional to wean down the dosage of the least necessary medications you may be taking. However, these seven pathways, when pursued with wisdom and common sense, create an additive synergistic effect. The more of these healing therapies that you can build into your life and routine, the more healthy you will become. You will increase in comfort, health, strength, happiness, energy, and longevity.

I have tried to provide enough variety in the techniques listed that there will be something for everyone. Some ideas require the assistance of a professional, some can be done alone, some are completely free, and others are expensive. Some require equipment, and some can be accomplished solely in your mind. Some require a single course of treatments, and others are a lifetime habit that you will enjoy for the rest of your days. So open your mind, open your heart, and begin to craft and brainstorm a plan to use the seven pathways of healing to change your life starting today.

You can be the hero of your own story. You can overcome the obstacles, scale the walls, and conquer the dragons in your life. You can become a hero to your family, friends, children, grandchildren, and generations to come by the decisions that you make, and the life that you create beginning now.

## Chapter 17 Action Steps

These Spiritual Pathway action steps are among the most critical in this book for your present and future happiness. Please take the time to write these out in your journal, a workbook, a note on your phone, or dictate it into an audio recording.

**Purpose Statement**- What is my life's purpose? Why am I here? What was I born to do?"

**Values Clarification Exercise**- Values are usually single words or short phrases such as: family, learning, financial success, contribution, adventure, creativity, etc. These are things that you value; that are most valuable to your life and happiness.

Brainstorm a list of 6-12 of values that are most important to you, then come up with a sentence, or short paragraph, that defines what that word means to you.

Then sequence these values in order of highest priority at the top of the list to lowest priority at the bottom.

Type out this list, print out several copies, and put them in various places around your home where you can read them often.

Consider how you invest your time and energy, and how much you are devoting to each value. Do your best to focus your most concentrated efforts toward your number-one value and less effort to your lowest value.

**Goals**- Brainstorm your list of goals that excite and motivate you. Decide on the chronological order of your goals, choose your most important 6-8 goals, and type them out. Post them in a prominent place where you can read over and visualize them daily.

**Legacy-**

- What sentence would you want written on your tombstone?
- What would you want to have said about you at your funeral?
- What do you want to be remembered for?
- What will you have accomplished by the end of your life?
- What relationships are most important to you in your life?
- Looking back, what charities did you start or contribute to?
- What causes did you champion?

**Gratitude**- Write out a list of at least 50 things that you are grateful for. Bonus points for going over 100 things.

Gratitude can be explored in the morning when you awake as a way to start your day off right, or at night in the form of a gratitude journal where you write out the specific things you are grateful for that day.

**Love, Service, Forgiveness**- Seek to make the Golden Rule, "Do unto others as you would have them do unto you", a guiding principle in your life. Meditate on who you love and who loves you, and seek to radiate unconditional compassion to all that you interact with.

Seek opportunities to get outside of yourself and serve others whenever you have the time and energy to do so.

Seek to forgive anyone who has hurt or offended you at any time in your life. You don't need to speak to them directly, you can just say to yourself "I forgive you, I release any anger, resentment, or frustration from my heart and I wish you the best in your life." You can forgive others even if they have passed away or you have lost contact with them.

**Faith**- Focus your mental energy on thoughts of faith, words of faith, and acts of faith. Seek out stories and connections with others who have overcome their cancer, or who have overcome a similar cancer to yours.

**Intuition**- What is one message that your higher self has been trying to tell you lately?

**Prayer**- If you believe in the power of prayer, then ask for the prayers and support of family and friends, and say personal prayers for your peace of mind and best outcome. Pray for others and their ultimate wellbeing.

**Other Spiritual Healing**- If you feel inspired to explore additional spiritual healing factors, you can learn more about the laying on of hands, shamanic journeys, chanting, or other countless healing methods. Pay close attention to your feelings and intuition so you can be led to the modalities that truly feel good to you.

## Reviews Save Lives

If you have enjoyed this book so far, and feel like it will help others as well, please take the time now to leave a quick star-rating or short review on Amazon or Goodreads. I sincerely believe that the application of the information in this book will be life-enhancing for every cancer patient or individual seeking cancer prevention. Every review counts and may help change or even save a life. Thank you in advance for your honest review, and for helping others learn more about this life-changing material.

# Chapter 18

## If You Undergo Surgery, Chemotherapy, Or Radiation

"Miracles happen everyday, change your perception of what a miracle is and you'll see them all around you."

–Bernie Siegel

First off, I just want to repeat that I absolutely support medical freedom for all. You should never be made to feel that a certain treatment is mandatory or required. Cancer is a disease that has many risks, and cancer treatments also come with many risks and side effects that can sometimes be as deadly as the cancer itself. As a patient or caregiver, it is imperative that you educate yourself about the risks and benefits of recommended treatments and their likelihood of extending your lifespan. Ask your oncologist questions until you fully understand the risks, benefits, and side effects of your treatment options.

If you are told that you have very low chances of survival, even with treatment, or that there are no available treatments for your situation, or if you just know that conventional treatments are not the path for you, then you can make the personal decision to work with your chosen team of health providers including: Naturopathic Doctors, Herbalists, Acupuncturists, Massage Therapists, Reiki Masters, Nutritional Health Coaches, etc to craft an amazing treatment plan based on the 7 Pathways that will work for your particular circumstances of personality, time, money, and energy.

If however, like the majority of patients, you decide to work with an oncologist for conventional treatments, then there are some incredible things you can do to help the chemotherapy to work even better at killing cancer cells, protect your normal cells, and dramatically reduce the side effects of the cancer treatments.

Oncologists are highly skilled and intelligent specialists, but they are human beings, and unless they choose to focus on integrative medicine self-education, then they have had almost zero education in the areas of nutrition, herbalism, physical therapy, hydrotherapy, or any of the other treatments outlined in the 7 Pathways. Don't let any doctor or other well-meaning person ever tell you that there is no evidence for natural or complementary therapies. This entire book is proof that there are mountains of evidence out there, it's just not what oncologists spend their free time reading about. Let oncologists be experts in surgery, chemotherapy, and radiation, and let natural health professionals be the experts in their own fields.

In other words, please don't ask your oncologist what you should eat to improve your cancer, or if this or that herb is safe for your cancer. They will most likely give you a blank stare, and say "eat whatever you want, just make sure you get plenty of calories." They have no training or experience in these areas, and they will most often shoot down your ideas as a knee-jerk response.

Tell your Doctor about the treatments you are interested in incorporating into your plan, but if they are not open to these ideas from the 7 Pathways, then it is your responsibility to keep looking for another oncologist until you find one that is open-minded, and that will respect you and your medical wishes.

These recommendations are a synthesis of the best practices from Naturopathic, Functional, and Chinese Medicine for healing and recovery after surgery, radiation, or chemo, and for increasing the effectiveness of chemotherapy and radiation therapies.

## Surgery

### Before:

**Discontinue Blood Thinning Supplements-** One week before surgery, stop taking: fish oil, garlic, ginger, enzymes, ginkgo, and vitamin E as these may interfere with successful surgical healing.

**Modified Citrus Pectin-** Pectasol 5g 3x per day -1 week before and 3 weeks after surgery.

**Vitamin C** - 1000 mg 3x daily.

**Immune Support**- Beta-glucans or medicinal mushroom blend, Echinacea angustifolia, Aloe vera juice

**Bone Broth**- as desired with meals.

**Any therapies from the Emotional Pathway**- to help with fear or anxiety about surgery

*If you are having surgery for breast cancer, and are still having a period, studies have shown there is better long-term survival if you schedule your surgery during the 2nd half of your cycle (day 15-28 after bleeding starts). This is because the estrogen that promotes cellular growth, and other molecules that promote angiogenesis, are lower in the 2nd half of the cycle.

**After-**

**Pain Medications**- ask your doctor about prescribing Tramadol instead of one of the other opiate pain medications (Oxycodone, Hydrocodone, Morphine, etc) because these commonly prescribed opiates can have immune-suppressing effects that we want to avoid when recovering from cancer surgery.

Topicals:

**Dr Christopher's Complete Tissue and Bone Ointment**- apply daily to any incisions after your stitches are removed for faster healing time and reduced scar formation.

**Arnica Ointment**- Apply as needed for pain or bruising.

**Essential Oils**- Possibilities include: Frankincense, Tea Tree, Helichrysum, Lavender, and Chamomile. For increased tissue healing, and decreased inflammation.

Internally:

**Modified Citrus Pectin**- 5 g 3x per day- for at least 3 weeks after surgery. (for 3 months after surgery is more ideal).

**Probiotics**- any refrigerated brand from a grocery or health food store- 2 caps with each meal for at least the 1st month after surgery.

**Proteolytic Enzymes**- Can help reduce inflammation, adhesions, and scar formation. As directed on the bottle.

**Whole-Food Multivitamin**- To ensure proper nutrients needed for healing.

**Dr Christopher's Complete Tissue and Bone Capsules**- 3 caps 3x per day until the bottle is done. This provides herbal nutrition for faster recovery.

**Herbs**- such as: Gotu Kola, Slippery Elm, Yarrow, & Calendula support tissue healing and reduced scar formation.

**Foods**- review the cancer-stem-cell killing foods list in the Molecular Pathway Part 1, and flood your system with these foods after surgery. Sometimes surgery can release these cancer stem cells into circulation and create micrometastases. These foods can help take out these survivors and stragglers.

## Radiation

**Before & During:**

**Fasting**- See the fasting chapter in the Physical Pathway if you need a quick review. This can powerfully weaken cancer cells in preparation for making radiation treatments even more effective.

Or

**Ketogenic Diet**- If you cannot do the 4-day fast option, you can do a plant-based keto diet for at least 1 week before and then during your radiation treatment window. See the food chapter if you need a quick review. This can powerfully weaken cancer cells in preparation for radiation treatments.

**Along with**

**Hyperthermia**- Hyperthermia is a type of cancer therapy that involves heating the body's tissues to temperatures ranging from

104-112 F (40-45°C) for a specified period of time. The heat can cause cancer cells to become more sensitive to radiation or chemotherapy, resulting in enhanced treatment outcomes. If you have a doctor that

uses a local hyperthermia machine, you can use that before going in for radiation treatment. If not, you can use the sauna in a local gym

for 20 min before each radiation session, or use a home tent Infra-red sauna for 30 min before each radiation treatment.

**Along with**

**Molecular Sensitizers**- This is a big category, so you can just pick 1 or 2 of the following herbs or supplements to internally support sensitizing the cancer cells to radiation, and protecting normal cells from radiation before, during, and after the radiation treatment window.

**Cod Liver Oil Capsules**- Contain natural vitamin E and Vitamin A that have both been shown to protect from radiation and improve immune status.

**Hydrogen Water**- A report stated that, "A randomized, placebo-controlled study showed that consumption of hydrogen-rich water reduces the biological reaction to radiation-induced oxidative stress without compromising anti-tumor effects." Hydrogen water is available in 2 main forms: either a machine that infuses hydrogen molecules into water, or as tablets you can dissolve into a water bottle with the lid on, and this diffuses the hydrogen into the water. This is an exciting supplement that has a growing body of research behind it.

**Mistletoe**- Available in liquid gemmotherapy (plant stem-cell) extracts, homeopathic preparations, or injected (Iscador, Helixor) versions.

**IV Hydrogen Peroxide or Ozone**- These treatments have been used by many alternative clinics to increase the oxygen content of the tissues, which is said to improve sensitivity to radiation and selectively harm cancer cells.

**Mushrooms**- Reishi, Turkey Tail, Poria, or Maitake D-Fraction have all been shown to help make radiation more toxic to cancer cells and support healthy cells.

**Quercetin**- 500 mg 3x per day

**Melatonin**- 10-20 mg each night before bed.

**Germanium**- is a trace element mineral that has been shown to improve NK cell activity, increase tissue oxygenation, and increase radiation sensitivity. The foods highest in germanium are shitake mushrooms, and garlic.

**All of the Following Herbs Have Been Studied to Support Making Radiation Therapy more Effective at Harming Cancer Cells and Also Protecting Normal Cells:**

Ashwagandha, Astragalus, Atractyloides, Barberry, Calamus, Calendula, Coptis, Eleuthero, Ginkgo, Ginseng, Goji Berries, GoldenSeal, Green Tea, Ligustrum, Milk Thistle, Oregon Grape, Remania, Rhodiola, Turmeric.

**After:**

You can continue any herbs you are taking for 1-2 years after the radiation treatments are ended. This may help mitigate the cancer-causing risks of radiation exposure. You can also rotate through these herbs for 2 months each, for a broader range of protective molecules.

**For Topical Radiation Burns**- pure Aloe Vera gel, or a spray bottle filled with the teas of slippery elm, calendula, lavender and 100% Aloe Vera juice.

**For Mouth Burns**- 1 scoop of glutamine powder with 1 teaspoon manuka honey dissolved in warm water then swished in the mouth for 5 minutes then spit out. Alternatively, you can use a special form of licorice root called DGL Solid Extract (Deglycyrrhizinated Licorice) available in lozenge or gel forms that can support oral tissue healing.

# Chemotherapy

**Concepts about the method, dosing, and timing of chemotherapy that can create better outcomes:** Ask your oncologist about, and encourage them to implement any of the following methods.

**Insulin Potentiated Chemotherapy (IPT)-** is a cancer treatment that involves the use of insulin to increase the effectiveness and reduce the side effects of chemotherapy. During IPT, insulin is given to the patient to lower their blood sugar levels, which causes cancer cells to become more receptive to chemotherapy drugs. Then, the patient is given a reduced dose of chemotherapy, which is more readily absorbed by the cancer cells due to their increased sensitivity and need for glucose.

**Chrono-chemotherapy-** is an approach to cancer treatment that involves administering chemo at specific times of the day based on the body's natural circadian rhythms. The idea behind this therapy is that the effectiveness of chemotherapies may be influenced by the body's internal clock, which can affect the way cancer cells respond to treatment. For example, some drugs may be more effective when administered during certain times of the day or night. In chrono-chemotherapy, the timing of chemotherapy administration is carefully planned to optimize drug effectiveness while minimizing side effects. This may involve taking into account factors such as the type of cancer, the patient's individual circadian rhythm, and the specific chemotherapy drugs being used.

**Fractionated Chemotherapy-** This approach involves dividing the total dose of chemotherapy drugs into smaller, more frequent doses over a longer period of time. The idea behind fractionated chemotherapy is to reduce the toxicity and side effects of chemotherapy while maintaining or improving treatment effectiveness. By giving smaller doses of chemotherapy over a longer period of time, healthy cells may have a chance to recover between treatments and reduce the risk of complications. The more conventional larger-dose or bolus chemotherapy is more convenient, but it can create more intense side effects.

**Before & During:**

This is the Same Concept As With Radiation- Pre-weakening the cancer cells by depriving them of easy fuel, by heat, and by molecular enhancers.

**Fasting-** See the fasting chapter in the Physical Pathway if you need a quick review. This can powerfully weaken cancer cells in preparation for making radiation treatments even more effective.

**Or**

**Ketogenic Diet-** If you cannot do the 4-day fast option, you can do a plant-based keto diet for at least 1 week before and then during your radiation treatment window. See the food chapter if you need a quick review. This can powerfully weaken cancer cells in preparation for radiation treatments.

**Along with**

**Hyperthermia-** Hyperthermia is a type of cancer therapy that involves heating the body's tissues to temperatures ranging from 104-112 F (40-45°C) for a specified period of time. The heat can cause cancer cells to become more sensitive to radiation or chemotherapy, resulting in enhanced treatment outcomes. If you have a doctor that uses a local hyperthermia machine, you can use that before going in for radiation treatment. If not, you can use the sauna in a local gym for 20 min before each radiation session, or use a home tent Infra-red sauna for 30 min before each radiation treatment.

**During:**

**Antioxidants-** Your Oncologist may have told you to avoid antioxidants during chemotherapy. Unfortunately, this is an old

wive's tale, and the more current research consistently shows that antioxidants have either a neutral or enhancing effect on

chemotherapy. You may need to educate your Oncologist on this point. The only exceptions to this that we know of are synthetic Beta-carotene and synthetic Vitamin E, both of which have been shown to increase cancer mortality, especially in smokers. However, these synthetic supplements should not be used by humans anyway so it's beside the point.

**Supplements That Have Been Shown To Enhance Chemotherapy-** Fish Oil, Melatonin, Quercetin, Vitamin D3, Vitamin E Succinate (especially with -platin drugs), Genistein (especially with Cisplatin), Theanine (especially with doxorubicin), Whey Protein Powder (especially with Methotrexate)

*Do not use quercetin if you treating colon cancer

**N-Acetyl Cysteine (NAC)- is a wonderful supplement that helps increase your body's internal antioxidant glutathione, but it is one supplement that may interfere with chemotherapy, **so avoid its use when in the active treatment phase.**

**Plants & Fungi That Have Been Shown To Enhance Chemotherapy & Protect Normal Cells-** Ashwagandha, Astragalus, Atractyloides, Black Currant Oil, Boswellia, Eleuthero, Goji Berries, Ligustrum, Maitake Mushroom, Milk thistle, Nutmeg, Pao Pereira, Poria Mushroom, Rehmannia, Reishi Mushroom, Turkey Tail Mushroom, Turmeric

**If You Develop Multiple Drug Resistance To Chemotherapy- These Herbs & Molecules Have Been Used To Block Chemo Drug Resistance In Cancer Cells-** Andrographis, Berberis, Campherol, Catharanthus, Coptis, Echinacea, Euphorbia, Genstein, Ginger, Graviola, Gynostemma, Jujubee, Licorice, Milk Thistle, Momordica, Phyllanthus, Polygonum, Poria Mushroom,

Quercetin, Rauwolfia, Remania, Rosemary, Salvia, Schisandra, Scutellaria, St John's Wort, Stephania, Turmeric.

**After:**

**Immune Enhancement- to increase white blood cell counts depleted by chemotherapy-** Astragalus, Echinacea, Ginseng, Ligustrum, Schizandra, all the medicinal mushrooms (Poria, Reishi, Turkey Tail, Shitake, Maitake, Chaga), Polyerga, and the Gemmotherapy (plant bud extract) Tamarix Gallica

**Tissue healing for GI upset, ulcers, or mucousitis-** Slippery Elm, Aloe Vera, Calendula, Marshmallow root powder, Chia seeds, Gotu Kola Powder, DGL Licorice Extract

**"Chemo Brain"** - Omega 3 Oils, CBD, Ginkgo biloba, Gotu Kola, Bacopa monnieri, Lion's Mane Mushroom, Acetyl-L-Carnitine, Neurofeedback Training, Acupuncture, Exercise.

**Nerve Pain-** Acetyl-LCarnitine, Alpha-Lipoic-Acid, B-complex, Blue Vervain, California Poppy, Co Q-10, Lion's Mane Mushroom, Melissa, Omega-3 Oils, Passionflower, Skullcap, Jamaican Dogwood, St John's Wort Oil (topically).

**To Prevent Heart Damage From Antitumor Antibiotics** (doxorubicin, mitomycin, etc)- Co-Q-10, Magnesium taurate, L-carnitine, D-ribose

After your final course of chemotherapy, it would be wise to ask your naturopathic or functional doctor to order a micronutrient test, (for example, Spectracell Micronutrient or Genova NutrEval) to assess what nutrients may have been depleted along your journey. You can then

supplement with these specific nutrients to fill in the gaps that have been created by the stresses of cancer treatment.

## Final Thoughts

As we conclude this portion of our journey together, I just want to thank you for your faith, trust, and perseverance. It takes determination to get to the end of a book like this, and I am so proud of the progress you have made.

If you have come to this point in the book, and you still feel like you need extra guidance and customization, I have a few openings to work with clients through telemedicine consultations worldwide. 6-month or 1-year programs are available to provide continued follow up and momentum on your personal healing path. If you would like more information, see http://RediscoverHealthNaturalMedicine.com.

Always remember that you are the hero of your own story, and you can take charge of the rest of your life with wisdom, poise, and happiness. I believe that one of the central purposes of life is to learn to be happy and to help others to be happy.

This is not just a shallow pleasure, but a true, deep, abiding, *joy* that comes from the inside out. By grabbing hold of your attention, and allowing you to reassess your priorities, cancer may be a gift from the universe. Life will end for all of us at some point; there is no way around this fact. So all we can do is live, learn, love, serve, and enjoy all the life that we are given.

Remember that the 7 Pathways are an upward spiral of health. As long as you maintain or grow your efforts to move forward along the emotional, physical, energetic, molecular, genetic, social, and spiritual pathways, you will vastly increase your probability of a long, happy, and healthy life.

May God bless you in your ongoing healing journey.

Dr David Lemmon

## Reviews Save Lives

If you have enjoyed this book, and feel like it will help others as well, please take the time now to leave a quick star-rating or short review on Amazon or Goodreads. I sincerely believe that the application of the information in this book will be life-enhancing for every cancer patient or individual seeking cancer prevention.

Every review counts, and may help to change, or even save, a life. Thank you in advance for your honest review, and for helping others to learn more about this life-changing material.

# Integrative Cancer-Treatment Centers

These Medical Centers follow many of the principles outlined in this book.

https://medericenter.org

https://www.envita.com

https://cancercenterforhealing.com

https://consultation.brio-medical.com

https://utopiacancercenter.com

https://www.immersionhealthpdx.com

https://www.lifeworkswellnesscenter.com

https://heal.hope4cancer.com

https://www.cancercenter.com

# If You Would Like Further Support

## The Biology of Hope: Community

For those who desire ongoing group support, Dr Lemmon has developed an online community where for only $47 per month you can access the entire video course version of this book as well as monthly live and on-demand group coaching and Q&A calls, resources, training videos, and a support community based around the information from this book.

For more information go to: https://rediscoverhealthnaturalmedicine.com

## The Biology of Hope: 6-Month Follow Up Program

If you desire more in-depth and personalized guidance with implementing the 7 Pathways of Healing in your life, the 6-month program is the perfect fit for you. You can meet one-on-one with Dr Lemmon over video conference once every month, with continued email support between visits. You will be able to customize your diet, mind-body medicine, supplements, and lifestyle to your personal situation, tastes, and genetics. Also included are 3 bonus 1-hour sessions for clinical hypnotherapy or counseling with a professional therapist.

For more information go to: https://rediscoverhealthnaturalmedicine.com

## The Biology of Hope: 12-Month Follow Up Program

If you feel like you need even more in-depth customized guidance for implementing the 7 Pathways of Healing Program, then the 12-month follow up program is the right fit for you. You will meet one-on-one with Dr Lemmon over a video consultation once every month, with continued email support between visits. You will be able to customize your diet, mind-body medicine, supplements, and lifestyle to your personal situation, tastes, and genetics. Also included are 6 bonus 1-hour sessions for clinical hypnotherapy or counseling with a professional therapist.

For more information go to: https://rediscoverhealthnaturalmedicine.com

# About The Author

Dr David Lemmon is a renowned naturopathic physician and author focused on healing cancer and other chronic conditions. He is an alumnus of National College of Natural Medicine in Portland, Oregon. His unique approach helps cancer patients increase their probability of a long-term remission while reducing the side effects of conventional treatments like: hair loss, nausea, pain, and fatigue.

He has a deep and abiding faith in the human body and its abilities to heal. You will never hear the words from him, "there's nothing more we can do for you".

He has advanced training in nutrition, herbal medicine, frequency medicine, and homeopathy. He has worked with thousands of patients throughout the country.

Through his 7 Pathways of Healing Program, people can live longer and live better. Dr Lemmon is author of *Natural Home & Herbal Healing*, and *Cancer & The Biology of Hope*.

Dr David and his wife are the proud parents of 6 children. He has a passion for teaching the principles of health, nature, and empowered living. When not working with patients, he enjoys painting, reading, movies, travel, cooking, martial arts, weight training, hiking, and camping.

www.ingramcontent.com/pod-product-compliance
Lightning Source LLC
LaVergne TN
LVHW061933070526
838199LV00060B/3832